WAR ON INFLUENZA 1918

HISTORY, CAUSES AND TREATMENT OF THE WORLD'S MOST LETHAL PANDEMIC

WAR HISTORY JOURNALS

"The single biggest threat to man's continued dominance on the planet is the virus."

— JOSHUA LEDERBERG

CONTENTS

INTRODUCTION

Pittsburgh was struck by an influenza epidemic in 1918. It first reared its ugly head late August in Boston. By early October, it was already spreading through the community of Pittsburgh. Though Pittsburgh saw the warning signs and took some necessary precautions to protect public health, the epidemic advanced viciously, leaving a high death toll in its wake.

Two military camps, holding a total of 7,000 soldiers, were stationed in Pittsburgh during the onset of the epidemic. The men were housed in makeshift barracks at camps located at the School of Technology in Carnegie and Pittsburgh University. These barracks had large dormitories for the soldiers to relax and mingle. Though ordinary sanitation arrangements were made, there was no opportunity for personal space, therefore the barracks were breeding grounds for disease. The first 2 cases of influenza were reported on October 2nd. There were four cases the next day, and eight cases on the following day.

The exponential growth rate of new cases meant that strict segregation and arrangements for the care of sick people had to be made. Military authorities took over part of the Elizabeth Steel Magee Hospital and prepared the wards for the coming epidemic. Major E. W. Day will forever be remembered for his quick thinking and clear leadership during the outbreak. His tireless work during the start of the epidemic was invaluable, and his firm quarantine regulations and the coordination of his medical forces helped contain the spread.

Working under Major E. W. Day's leadership, Capt. H. H. Hendershott took charge of the hospital's management, which was pushing its capacity limit at the time. Within 6 days, the 150-bed hospital housed more than 300 influenza patients. Provisions for new cases had to be made, and on October 5th, Pittsburgh University granted the military access to its medical school's lab facilities. Originally, it was planned that only essential laboratories would be used for patient care. However, as the epidemic spread, the Medical School closed and gave the Military Hospital control of all laboratory facilities.

This established the departments of pathology, clinical microscopy, physiology, physiologic-chemistry, and bacteriology. These dedicated people worked tirelessly for a span of five weeks, by which time the epidemic was losing power as fewer new cases were being reported. The laboratory work of the Military Hospital ended on November 9th.

Mercy Hospital was another contributor to the aid of the influenza epidemic. The hospital provided more than 100 beds to care for those who could not be accommodated by the Military Hospital. Unfortunately, with so many cases suddenly thrown at the army's medical staff, it was impossible for them to give in-depth detailed reports. It was just as hard for the medical officers, who were transferred to new posts throughout the course of the epidemic, to give clear reports on the work done at the Military Hospital. That being said, the clinical findings at Mercy Hospital and those at other hospitals still show remarkable parallels. Since the research carried out during the epidemic was as intensive as it could be, the workers involved agree that they would be better prepared if another similar plague were to strike again.

In the early days of the influenza outbreak, director of Singer Memorial Laboratory, Dr. S. R. Haythorn, became interested in protecting people against infection. At the time there were many claims of the kind of immunity that vaccinations could provide. Dr. Haythorn began preparing the necessary materials, hoping to gain positive results from these vaccines. The value of his work was seen in time, as the outbreak was once again losing traction.

BRIEF HISTORY OF INFLUENZA

INSPIRED BY THE WORK OF JAMES I. JOHNSTON, M. D.

Influenza dates back to the early Christian Era of the Middle Ages. That being said, it wasn't until 1510 that the first epidemic was reported. It was the first reliable record of the influenza virus as we know it today. A few things stood out in the report, most notably the severity in which the disease attacked pregnant women, and the presence of pneumonia and nose bleeds in the infected. In 1580, it was also reported that influenza had a tendency to come back after remaining dormant for a brief time. It would ramp up in August and September and become more aggressive and likely to cause pneumonia in October and November. The summer of 1657 was rather warm, but winter hit hard and early, that spring was notably humid, and an outbreak of influenza struck London in April 1658.

Popular opinion at the time said that the weather influenced the body's circulation. It was believed that this poisoned the blood, and that is what caused people to fall ill. The influenza virus thrived in big cities and continued to return each year. In 1675, the term "tussis epidemicus" was used for the disease because of its effects on pregnant women.

Fall in England, 1676 started off mild, but the weather turned cold and moist without warning, good breeding grounds for influenza. Germany was also suffering during this time. In 1693, a bad influenza epidemic struck Dublin. Attention was called to a specific characteristic of this epidemic. That age greatly impacted one's reaction to the infection. At the time, this seemed like a unique characteristic.

The winter of 1728 was strong throughout Europe, that spring was cold and the weather during summer and fall fluctuated. The weather was again a factor in the epidemic of 1732, and this outbreak was one of the longest and most relentless, extending up to 1737. Despite this, the mortality rate in 1733 for people other than infants and the elderly hit an all-time low. The weather was highly variable, and there was abundant thick fog throughout the duration of the epidemic. During the outbreak, it was also noticed that people in the isolation of prisons and hospitals were less likely to be affected by the influenza virus.

The next epidemic took place from 1742 to 1743. The weather was intense once again, and the disease spread across Europe. It is thought that the now-common term "influenza" was first used during this epidemic. During this time, England had rather mild cases, but Southern Europe had a much rougher time, with more severe cases being reported. Oddly enough, weather conditions during this outbreak were mild and dry, which prompted skepticism over how much the weather and air quality really influenced the disease. It was also reported that relapses often occurred if a patient was exposed to the disease soon after the initial infection. Such relapses were often more severe than the first time.

The epidemic of 1762 followed a period of variable cold and moist weather, and it spread across Europe. Then, in Germany, 1775, an epidemic began after a warm, mild spring, and it once again spread across Europe. This event reinforced the idea that the disease was not caused by changing weather patterns. During the strong presence of the disease in 1775, concerns were raised around the opinion that weather conditions were not responsible for the spread of influenza. The cause for the spread was unknown. In 1780, the disease began in France after dramatically alternating weather, and it went on to spread around the world. Then, in 1782, Russia experienced a sudden 40-degree shift in temperature, and nearly 4,000 people fell ill with the influenza virus. It was another world-spanning epidemic. During this time, the discovery was made that influenza was spread by close contact with a sick person. It was theorized that there could be asymptomatic carriers of the disease.

The influenza epidemic struck America hard in 1789. It plagued the country from September to December and popped up again in the spring. Even the president fell gravely ill with the virus. It had struck Paris and Vienna the year prior and hit Russia by the end of 1799. Next came the epidemic of 1802, which lasted 6 months. Pneumonia was not as common during this epidemic, but it was especially dangerous to pregnant women.

In 1810, the virus engulfed much of China and Manila, and it was found that similar illnesses were also plaguing animal populations during that time. During the 1833 epidemic, it was found that animals, most notably horses, could be affected by the disease as well. We now call the diseases that spread between animals and people zoonotic diseases. They have been linked to a number of brutal disease outbreaks. Influenza was strongly linked to other epidemics for the first time in 1837. It would either precede, follow or replace other epidemics.

Mild epidemics followed in the years between 1846 and 1875. There was some confusion for doctors during this time, as it was hard to distinguish between cerebrospinal meningitis and influenza. Some even believed that they were the same disease, only in differing severities. The American Medical Association eventually started a committee to make investigations into the diseases to help settle this division of opinions among doctors.

The outbreak of 1889 was a true pandemic. Children and the elderly had the highest mortality rate during this epidemic. Males accounted for the most deaths, partly due to the fatigue of work. This pandemic was believed to have started in Asia, as so many others had, and from there spread around the globe. The disease spread rapidly, affecting roughly 40% of the world's population. It then disappeared just as fast several weeks later. Improvement in transportation surely had a direct correlation to the way in which this epidemic spread. This close connection was further proven by the fact that large cities were hit first, followed by smaller cities, in the fact that railroad towns had more outbreaks than isolated villages.

The question whether influenza spreads outwards in all directions like spilled water, or if it can leap from place to place, was eventually settled by congress when they learned it does both. There was a growing concern about whether the influenza virus spread faster than other viruses. Especially after people learned how it could easily move from the mucous membrane into the air by coughing or sneezing.

Also, the fact that people could carry and spread the disease for a few days without knowing it before they began to feel ill. Adding to the concern was how it could affect people of any age. It could live on surfaces and be transferred by merchandise. It could spread short distances through the air.

Following the 1891 pandemic, there were several outbreaks in America and England. There were oddly no cases in Germany or France, despite travelers from England and America. Because of this, people started to wonder if the French and Germans were somehow more immune to Influenza. However, the slow development of these particular outbreaks had more to do with this case than immunity levels. That being said, the world's population has become less susceptible to the disease over time and continues to do so as more time passes. This increase in human immunity to a virus is now called "herd immunity," and it happens with each new persistent pandemic.

Though there had been no proven connection to the seasons, by 1889, there was a clear pattern of the disease striking in the fall or spring and becoming dormant during summer. This meant that it could confidently be said that influenza was not impacted by specific weather conditions. But by the consistency of the seasons. It had two geographic presentations: the pandemic stage, which means worldwide or wide-spreading, and the endemic stage, which refers to more local and constant prevalence.

It was also proven that the disease was easily spread by direct or close contact. There had been numerous cases of people traveling abroad and returning with the virus, only to spread it to their family, which then spread to their community, and so on. Even the most isolated parts of the world that had not previously been exposed to the virus suffered outbreaks that were started by outsiders. These unfortunate events allowed for more study into the spread and decline of epidemics, and led to a better understanding of influenza. By this time, the virus was hardly ever life-threatening, and the mortality rate continued to decline.

THE 1918 EPIDEMIC

On August 28, 1918, the Boston Naval Station was struck with 50 cases of influenza, which became more than 2,000 in the next two weeks. Roughly 5% of cases developed broncho-pneumonia, and the mortality rate was more than 60%. It quickly spread to Camp Devens and by November there were 3,339 civilian cases in Boston. The epidemic hit New York in September. The peak of the outbreak was in October, and by December there were 136,061 cases. There were 11,725 reported influenza deaths and 11,601 more deaths due to pneumonia. The virus also hit Pittsburgh hard during October, with a terrifying rate of nearly 600 new cases being reported daily between October 16th to October 28th. From October and December, there were 23,268 reported cases in Pittsburgh and roughly 2,052 deaths linked to pneumonia.

The first warning of the Spanish flu in America was sent out in July 1918. It was recognized in the public by September, and many cases included pneumonia. This is when it was first advised to isolate patients, and for care providers to wear masks. Patients remained in isolation for

10 days after recovery to protect them from relapse. People were warned against coughing, sneezing, spitting, and gathering in large crowds. Churches, theaters, and other public places were closed in October, and funerals became strictly private affairs.

Colleges were another area hit hard by the epidemic. Pennsylvania's Bryn Mawr College had 465 students, and there were a total of 110 student cases either on campus or at home. Wellesley College had 1,593 students, with roughly 545 cases reported and only one death. Harvard, with 3,193 suffered at least 227 cases and 5 deaths. Princeton, with 1,050 students, had around 70 cases and one related death. Yale was hit particularly hard, with 2,265 students, Yale had a staggering 1,013 cases and 249 deaths from pneumonia.

There was a grand total of roughly 675,000 American deaths linked to the Spanish flu epidemic of 1918. After the epidemic, there was a weather comparison of 12 major American cities. Remarkably, they all had fair weather during the outbreak. This once again points not to specific weather as a factor in the disease, but rather the consistent seasonal pattern. We now know that the flu does follow a seasonal pattern, worsening from fall to spring and becoming inactive during summer.

* * *

For a long time, people failed to see that what they thought were several diseases turned out to be one, now known as influenza. At the time, the influenza virus was the single most pervasive, widespread disease. It lasted for years with gaps of time between each major epidemic. Most cases of pneumonia during this time were eventually linked to influenza, and that pneumonia was a factor in most of the deaths of the disease. Specific weather conditions were not responsible for the spread of the disease, though influenza did follow a seasonal pattern. The spread was caused by close contact with the sick, as well as by respiratory droplets from sick people that spread only short distances through the air or that got on surfaces.

With the advancements in modern life, the disease was able to spread faster than any virus before it. With faster transportation methods, more international travel, and larger populations, the influenza virus thrived. It started out with a high mortality rate and affected a larger portion of the world's population than previous pandemics could. Luckily, the virus weakened over time as the human population as a whole grew more immune to the disease. The influenza virus continued to impact people, and take lives, but it is no longer the highly deadly disease that it was at its start.

The 1918 influenza epidemic and those preceding it will forever mark an important time in medical history. Influenza was a disease unlike anything that had come before it, and with its many struggles came revolutionary medical work and a better understanding of the nature of epidemics. With the epidemics came temporary hospitals and labs that would not have existed without the existence of such a disease. The work done at these temporary sites was later carried on by permanent hospitals, labs, and medical schools for further medical research.

Two very distinct and comparable groups admitted to the Mercy Hospital provided some of the most valuable clinical observations. The first group was made up of 153 soldiers ages 18 to 23. The second group was made up of 394 civilians of varying ages, from super young to the elderly. In the first group, patients came in as soon as they were aware they had the disease. Patients in the second group usually came in only after they had already been sick for several days with headaches, body aches, and loss of appetite, along with other symptoms and pneumonia in some cases. This provided a strong study group of both young healthy people who were admitted early and typically suffered less, and others who may be old or young and who often suffer more, in part because of age, but also because they were already very sick upon arrival to the hospital.

INCUBATION TIME AND DURATION

The incubation period, or the amount of time between when a person is first exposed to a disease to when they show the first symptoms has been a source of fascination and debate since the first detection of its existence by the medical and scientific communities. For example, say a farmer from a community without any influenza cases traveled to the city. He was exposed to the disease by sitting in the same seat on the train that a sick person with a cough had previously sat in. Roughly forty-eight hours later, he began experiencing the first noticeable symptoms of influenza. Soon, his wife started showing symptoms, and within two days their child fell ill as well. The farmer became sick the moment he sat on the train, and his family became sick the moment they were in close contact with him, but they didn't start showing symptoms until the disease had completed its incubation period.

The scary thing is that the disease, like so many, affected people differently. Say a young healthy man was infected with the influenza virus. He continued to spread the disease

unknowingly during the incubation period before his symptoms started. Then, he began to feel mild symptoms, but
because the symptoms were so mild, he continued to go
about his life until finally falling ill enough to stay home. He
makes a full recovery but has spread the disease to an
elderly man who develops a much more serious case of
influenza. With the same virus responsible for the mild case
in the young man, the old man falls violently ill and is
hospitalized. He later died of complications from pneumonia brought on by the influenza virus. This shocking
example shows how the incubation period of a disease like
influenza is directly tied to the impact epidemics have on
the population, and should never be overlooked.

The communicability, or ease of spread between people,
is another key aspect of diseases such as influenza. A strong
example of this was in a house where a member lay ill with
a bad case of influenza in a sick room. He was separated
from the rest of the house for several weeks. Other members
of the house passed the door to the sick room daily, yet they
did not catch the disease. This strongly suggested that
influenza, despite being transmittable by close contact, was
not a true airborne disease. This meant that it did not travel
long distances through the air, and this fact was reassuring
to many people.

The duration of the disease is another important factor
in its severity. In the case of the influenza virus, it has a
duration of several days on average. Because soldiers who
fell ill in the barracks were easily monitored, they served as
a valuable study group to learn more about influenza and its
duration. It is important to note that these soldiers were
young and fairly healthy prior to falling ill. The average
duration of influenza within this group was 6 to 7 days, with

the shortest recorded duration being a day, and the longest being 10 days. As for reported civilian influenza cases, the average duration was between 4 and 6 days, with females showing longer durations on average. The longest reported duration in the civilian population was 16 days.

DIFFERENT FORMS OF INFLUENZA

The influenza virus can best be described as a variable, as it has several forms. Influenza epidemics of the past helped classify influenza as either the respiratory form, gastro-intestinal form, circulatory form, psychic form, renal form, nervous form, or other. The forms were classified based on the symptoms of different patients. Headache, body aches, loss of appetite are common symptoms of influenza, and so are respiratory symptoms. In some cases, lower respiratory issues arose early in the illness. These cases were the most likely to be fatal. Nausea, vomiting and diarrhea, specific kinds of psychosis, were rarely the leading symptoms. Because of this, it is the respiratory form of the influenza virus that is best known in the medical community. Arising from the respiratory form, two distinct forms of the virus were recognized.

The first form of influenza is the upper respiratory form. This form involves the trachea and larger bronchi. It accounted for roughly 52-60% of all influenza cases. The primary symptoms in these cases were a sore throat and cough. Other than acute bronchitis, there were no deep chest symptoms. The upper respiratory form of influenza is a simple form with a few serious complications. This means that the patients often have a less severe case of influenza with this form.

The second form of influenza is the lower respiratory or deep chest form. The symptoms of this form are very similar to those of bronchiolitis or broncho-pneumonia. There is often fluid buildup in the lungs, which often leads to pneumonia. There were a few cases of lower respiratory influenza that acted a lot like labor pneumonia. Unfortunately, this caused much confusion as it was often hard to distinguish between the two.

Along with the influenza virus came the fever. As the body fights off the infection, the core temperature rises. It was not uncommon for influenza patients to experience a sudden fever of 102–104 degrees Fahrenheit. The fever typically lasted several days before beginning to subside. Once the fever broke, the patient could rest assured that they were on the path to recovery. That is, so long as the fever didn't spike again, and no serious complications had appeared during that time. However, this wasn't always the case. There were cases in which one's fever would drop a degree or two, only to rise again in the following days.

In cases where the fever spiked for a second time, Cyanosis often followed. This meant that a high for too many days in a row could indicate serious lung issues. A high fever that persisted for more than five days often meant that the lungs were filling with fluid. Patients would notice a bluish discoloration in their hands and feet as their bodies struggled to get enough oxygen. These were the most serious cases.

Interestingly enough, the heart rate was hardly affected by the presence of such fevers. Even if a patient was gravely ill, their pulse often remained strong and healthy. For the most part, patients' pulse rate stayed between 84 to 96. This was surprising, especially in cases with serious complications. Even the sickest of patients tended to have a healthy pulse. It wasn't until just before a sick patient died that their pulse would spike for the first time.

Similarly, the respiration rate in patients remained normal until complications arose. For the duration of the disease, most patients could breathe normally. That is, unless they suffered from more serious lung complications. Breathing became more difficult after the lungs started filling with fluid, or other complications began. As the complications started, the respiratory rate would increase. Unfortunately, this increase was often the first sign of a very difficult road for the patient. Many patients who suffered from respiratory complications would ultimately end up dying.

The relationship between the pulse rate and the respiration rate was even more interesting. It would be reasonable to assume that the pulse would increase as the respiratory rate increased. After all, the struggle for oxygen puts a huge strain on the body. However, this was not the case for most patients. Even when the respiratory rate accelerated, the pulse rate often remained slow and stable.

There was one case of influenza that lasted seven days. This seemed like a fairly simple case. However, the patient's breathing soon became rapid due to lung issues. Despite this, the pulse rate remained at a steady 96. The patient eventually died from respiratory complications, most likely fluid in the lungs. Her breathing became increasingly rapid. This gave way to only agonal breaths during the last moments of her life. Remarkably, the patient's heartbeat stayed consistent throughout this. Despite fighting for oxygen, her heartbeat never wavered until the very moment in which she died.

There were always exceptions. Many cases showed pulse and respiratory rates as separate, but this wasn't always the case. Both the pulse and respiratory rate would increase together in some cases. In other cases, they would increase without any warning or sign of serious complications. This only adds to the many variants of the influenza virus.

Early in the epidemic, pale skin was noticed on the faces of the sick. At the time, belladonna poisoning was a common occurrence. The flushed faces of those affected by influenza looked very similar to those suffering from poisoning. A flushed face was one of the first signs that a person was sick, and a strong indicator that the lungs were being affected. It could even be an indicator of cyanotic, or fluid-filled lungs.

When cyanosis was first recognized in cases, it was often hard to see the changes in the lungs. That is, other than acute bronchitis, which was more easily identified. Soon, more clear signs appeared. Cyanosis was first seen in the face. It then appeared as bluish discoloration of the hands. It was often compared to the cyanosis sometimes caused by the overuse of certain coal tar derivatives. In fact, more deaths may have occurred from these prescriptions than from influenza-related deaths.

In cyanotic cases, neither blood nor hemoglobin was found in the urine of patients. Nose bleeds were sometimes present and were later linked to cyanosis. A few patients even suffered from coughing up blood. In these cases, there was always fluid buildup in the lungs. Cyanosis was common at the time. It was primarily found in cases of lobar pneumonia. However, influenza-related cyanosis was differ-ent. It struck early on, and without visible signs of lung trouble. It also tended to disappear once clear lung complications were visible. It was not linked to a disruption of the circulatory system. The pulse of patients remained steady, and it wasn't linked to fluid in the lungs. It is also worth noting that patients with cyanotic influenza also saw a drop in blood pressure.

The dramatic difference from influenza-related cyanosis and other causes of cyanosis led to much confusion. Attempting to control the disease, doctors used circulatory stimulants that were typically used to help treat cyanosis. However, this had little impact on the influenza virus. This led to a desperate last resort. The use of oxygen. At first, this seemed like it was working. However, the positive results didn't last. In the end, there wasn't much difference in outcomes between cases with and without the use of oxygen.

In the first stages of influenza, white blood cell numbers fell. They had a hard time increasing after this drop in number. Their numbers hardly increased as the infection attacked the lungs. There is no clear explanation of why this sudden leukopenia occurred. Some thought that infection came on so suddenly with influenza that the body had no time to properly react. Others believe that it is simply a strange toxic blood reaction to the virus. In the end, it was left as just a strange characteristic of the influenza disease.

One of the first symptoms reported by patients was a feeling of increased weakness. This symptom often began before a spike in temperature or any other early symptom. This feeling of weakness had also been reported in previous epidemics. However, in these cases, the weakness was not a clear early symptom. That being said, this symptom remains important in recognizing the disease.

One example of this was the story of one young soldier

inflicted with the virus. He woke up early as usual and began getting ready. While doing some light exercises, he noticed a slight feeling of fatigue. He became extremely weak only a few hours later. Upon hearing of this, medical officers called him. They found that he had a low fever, and he was ordered to bed. This was the first sign that the soldier was battling invisible influenza invaders. This was just one of many similar cases.

As with so many aspects of influenza, the cases with lung complications added to the confusion. This is especially true if one does not understand pathology. With no clear uninformed opinions, the debates surrounding the nature of the infection led to very little useful insight. There were numerous reports made on influenza. However, they shared contradicting information. By this time, it was clear that no two groups could agree on the bacteriology and pathology of the epidemic. With so much uncertainty, many were hesitant to speak with any resolution about the disease.

Despite the confusion, it could still be said that the lower respiratory tract was greatly impacted. The cases that involved the lungs and lower respiratory tract that were the most severe. These cases were a good portion of all cases. Roughly 40-50% of cases developed pneumonia. During this time there remained some doubts and questionable diagnosis. However, other symptoms came together to indicate influenza in many cases. The physical description of these influenza cases shows why there was doubt.

It is important to note the general condition of the patient at the first sign of lung complications. Patients who were thought to have a simple case of influenza often worsened with time. They may start out with slight bronchitis or tracheitis and be a little pale or bluish. This led to a fever that was longer than the typical 3-7 days. Localized pain would begin in the chest as the respiration rate increased. This often pointed to an internal chest lesion. The lungs would continue to get worse as they filled with fluid. As the virus worsened, lesions could appear in one of the lower lobes of the lungs. These lesions could then spread along the interlobar sulcus, or down the spinal column. The lesions could be found in small areas, or they could connect and form one giant lesion. In some cases, the lesions healed on their own. However, the lesions stubbornly remained in other cases.

In many cases involving lung complications, patients would cough up foul material. This could contain blood and yellowish-green chunks of puss-like matter. The matter was accompanied by watery fluid or frothy mucus. The amount of matter coughed up was rarely much. That being said, there were cases with excessive amounts of coughed-up matter. At times, it could also be very thick and aggravating to the patient.

The symptoms were very similar to broncho-pneumonia. Within a few hours to a day, the lower lobes of the lungs would begin to become rigid. One distinguishing factor of influenza-related pneumonia was the presence of a small, consistently clear section. Another key symptom was the crackling, vesicular breathing. If the patient made it to the recovery stage, they may still have a long road. In many cases, the recovery time stretched over several weeks. One pathologist soon contradicted the idea of only lower lobe lesions being present. It was found that there were lesions present in all lobes in a staggering 65% of all influenza cases. This was explained away by saying that the pathology in the upper lobes must have been ineffective or insufficient.

Surprisingly, the physically noticeable pathology was

not the key indicator of the outcome. It was the general infections or toxins in the blood that gave more information about the possible outcome. These signs could only be partially noticed in the respiratory system. These factors also had a direct impact on the success rate of various treatment methods. It was not uncommon for patients to die before going through all the typical stages of pneumonia. If they had lived longer, their lung pathology would be easier to see and understand. This would be easier to treat than the spongy cyanotic lung tissue often present in influenza cases.

One of the typical physical signs doctors could often use was body temperature. This was not the case with influenza, as the patient's temperature was often inconsistent. The temperature could stay elevated for several days without any clear chest signs. It may then start to fall in a typical manner. It was at this time that clear chest signs showed up, either slowly or suddenly. The temperature could then remain consistent for the remainder of the illness while one or both lungs stayed rigid. There were some cases in which the temperature fell drastically without any clear chest signs being present. The separate body temperature and chest signs only added to the difficulty of the disease.

In one case, two strong healthy men came in with signs of pneumonia, but no signs of solidification in the lungs. Within 12 hours, both patients experienced a dramatic drop in temperature. The physicians were surprised to find solidification in both lower lung lobes. This solidification was thought to have occurred during the time in which the patients' temperatures fell. Both men recover, but at a slow pace. If the patients got up too soon, their lungs could be impacted again. Because of the irregular symptoms of influenza, the diagnosis was extremely difficult. Physicians had to forget what they thought they knew about pneumonia and learn how pneumonia caused by influenza reacted in the body.

Adding to the difficulties, labs gave very little assistance. This was especially true at the beginning of the epidemic. This was partially due to the insufficient number of lab workers. In addition, the unusual lab results for influenza were difficult to understand. Since the labs provided little insight, doctors turned to other tactics. X-rays were one tactic to examine the chest. Unfortunately, X-rays were not available for every case. Even in the cases that used X-rays, the strange lesion patterns were difficult to interpret despite the health professionals' best efforts. There were also cases in which the patient was so sick that it was best to disturb them as little as possible.

In the end, it was shown that X-rays were not the best method of examination. That being said, they were a lot better than nothing. X-rays were not helpful in diagnosing the full extent of the disease, or in aiding the understanding of acute cases. That being said, they proved incredibly valuable in cases with complications or delayed recovery.

DIAGNOSING INFLUENZAL
PNEUMONIA

A clear diagnosis can eventually be found for even the most confusing of diseases. It takes time, reflection on the past, reliable lab tests, a thorough physical exam, and intelligent thinking. The road may be long, but the effort will be worth it in the end. Influenza was a baffling disease for physicians in its time. At the time, influenzal pneumonia was best known for its bacteriology, pathological changes, and physiological disturbances. The main way to identify and diagnose it was by looking at the history of the disease. This was true for both mild and severe cases. Now, thanks to years of hard work, Influenza is well understood. It is commonplace in our lives and most don't think twice about it. We have vaccines to fight it, and it hardly affects normal life anymore.

As influenza became more well known, it became clear that it impacted the respiratory tract. It also became clear that any pulmonary disturbance could hint at coming influenzal pneumonia. A steady temperature, cough, cyanosis, slow pulse, weakness, or drop in white blood cells could help diagnosis more than chest signs. Influenza was separated from bronchitis and broncho-pneumonia in diagnosis due to its more severe nature. It was separated from other lung infections in diagnosis due to the drop in white blood cells. It was also separated from croupous pneumonia because of its more confusing symptoms. The separation of influenzal pneumonia from acute tuberculosis proved to be more difficult, especially if there is no reliable history available. The best differentiation between the two was the fact that pulmonary tuberculosis typically began in the upper lungs whereas influenzal pneumonia began in the lower lobes. The presence or lack of tuberculosis causing bacteria in the mucus was the ultimate differentiation factor.

Lesions in cases with heavy lung involvement hardly ever provide a culture of pure Pfeiffer bacteria. In many cases, these bacteria were nonexistent. In their place were micro-organisms, including pneumococcus and streptococcus. These organisms are commonly found in pneumonia patients. That begs the question, are all influenza cases with heavy lung involvement simply complications of the disease? It could be that Pfeiffer bacteria cause lesions and prepare the tissue for the invasion of other germs commonly found in other forms of pneumonia. This meant that lesions commonly found in the lung were classified as part of influenza. Lesions found elsewhere were classified as complications.

The most common complication of influenza is tied to the pleural membranes. Pneumonia typically starts in the chest with localized pain. In the case of influenza, the microorganisms responsible for these things run wild. They do not follow a typical path of infection. This helps explain why the complications seem to vary so widely. There were many cases in which fluid in the lungs was suspected. This was often not the case because the confusing physical signs were easily misinterpreted.

Following the pneumonia outbreak of 1918, it was assumed that there would be many cases of fluid or abscesses in the lungs. Again, this was not the case. There was only one reported case with persistent fluid in the lungs and only one known case with lung abscesses. This low number of cases seemed strange and may not have accurately depicted reality. This suspicion was later confirmed when several other hospital reports were shown to have multiple cases of both fluid and abscesses present in the lungs. One case stood out from the rest. The patient was admitted twice with localized chest pain and suspicion of lung discharge. X-ray examinations pointed to fluid in the lungs, but no fluid was found with the needle test. Roughly eight weeks later, pus was found in the left lung. This was just one of many such influenza cases. Once again confirming the difficulty in understanding and diagnosing the disease.

In some cases, the swelling was noticed from the pharynx to the trachea. It was intense enough to cause labored breathing and abundant mucus and pus discharge. The lungs themselves remained clear, but the patients were in danger of dying from these complications. Similar complications included a handful of sinus infections, mild ear infections, and antrum disease. In epidemics prior to this, there were additional reported complications. This included tonsillitis and mastoiditis. Once again it was proven that the lower respiratory tract was more severely impacted than the upper respiratory tract.

Unlike some other infections, the kidneys remained

unaffected by the infections caused by influenza. The protein of albumen was found in the urine, but there was no evidence that the kidneys were inflamed. Another interesting reaction was that of the muscles. While in recovery, one patient was reported with sudden pain developing in the hip that attended to his lower back and thigh. This brought on the suspicion that he had developed pus abscess. After several tests came back negative, there was nothing he could do but rest. The pain turned out to be a benign muscle reaction, and he eventually made a full recovery.

Osteitis or the swelling of the bone was also found in some cases. This was typically seen in the vertebrae. The swelling led to incredible suffering before some patients eventually died. An investigative autopsy was never done on the first reported case. After this, another patient suffering from the same thing was thought to have Pott's disease. A plaster cast was applied to the patient, and his condition improved enough for him to leave the hospital. There was a great hesitation to link the microorganisms responsible for influenza to these bone lesions. That is, until a case was reported that showed clear links between the two. The case was of a 16-month-old child. The child had localized bone disease in the upper tibia. An incision was made to the inflamed area, and pus was found. A smear test of this pus confirmed that it contained the same bacteria responsible for influenza B.

Transient glycosuria is perhaps one of the most interesting influenza complications. The first patient suffering from this complication was a middle-aged woman who was having trouble with her vision. Mild inflammation of the optic nerve was found on closer examination. Upon finding this, doctors ran tests on the patient's urine. It was found that she had an excess of sugar in her urine. This problem was solved by decreasing her carbohydrate intake. Slowly, she regained her vision. It took nearly a month for her symptoms to disappear and her vision to return to normal. Similar cases had been found following previous influenza epidemics, though some cases had no vision impairment.

RISK OF PREGNANCY

Though it was obviously not a complication of influenza, pregnancy could directly impact the severity of the virus. There was a study done on five pregnant women who had fallen ill with influenza. The mothers were more than likely scared for their baby's safety as well as their own. Doctors and nurses were short-handed, and the mothers were sent to the Obstetrical Department once complications arose. This department made up for the short supply of health care providers, and they did great work while caring for influenza patients. Three of the pregnant women went into early labor or had miscarriages. One woman sadly died from complications. The other two delivered healthy babies and made a full recovery.

The two women who delivered healthy babies and recovered were lucky. Most pregnant women who get influenza were in grave danger. It was likely that pregnant women would lose their baby during the worst of the virus regardless of how far along they were. In a study of 50 pregnant women, 42% lost their baby. These women also had a less likely chance of recovering than women who were not pregnant. Even if their labor was uninterrupted, pregnant women had roughly a 48% higher chance of dying than other women. If the woman went into labor or miscarried, she had a startling 80% chance of dying. If a pregnant woman developed pneumonia during the influenza virus, her chances of survival were even slimmer.

There are a few theories of why women with influenza often miscarry or go into early labor. One is that carbon-dioxide levels in the blood could cause contractions strong enough to prompt labor to begin. Another theory is that toxins from the infection kill the unborn baby, which is then rejected by the body. This was most likely to happen when the fetus was still immature. There were also several theories as to why the mothers would die shortly after losing a baby. One theory was that they died simply because of the shock of labor. Another theory was that labor increased the carbon dioxide levels in the blood, which overwhelmed the already stressed respiratory system. Other theories included death from hemorrhaging, a sudden decrease in abdomen pressure, and added strain on the heart. Whatever the reason, it became clear that influenza during pregnancy was a grim diagnosis.

It is often hard to tell if symptoms that arise after one has been affected by influenza are complications of the disease itself, or if they are the result of sequelae. In other words, it can be difficult to tell complications of influenza apart from separate infections that arise after influenza has run its course. It would almost seem that influenza had a dormant period in which it was present in the body but showed few symptoms. This is because recovered influenza patients, free from influenza, could still show new symptoms. These symptoms could persist for a very long time, developing separately from the original infection. These infections were eventually defined as sequelae infections since they followed the original influenza virus.

One such infection was chronic bronchitis or a tubercular lesion. These cases were hard to understand, and they caused much confusion. It was often unclear if the lesions were due to a recent influenza illness, or if it existed before the person became ill. It was also frequently hard to tell if it had originated from pneumococci, streptococci, or tuberculous bacteria. In confusing cases such as these, medical professionals often look to past illnesses to help them form a diagnosis.

Perhaps most useful in making a diagnosis was the physical exam. This would give doctors more insight into where the lesions were located. From here, they could more accurately determine whether the lesions began before the current influenza infection. If the lesions are found solely towards the top of the lungs, it is probably a previous or separate case of tuberculous. If the lesions are found near the base of the lungs, they are most likely due to influenza. With that being said, it was still common to confuse tuberculosis with post influenza symptoms. This was a source of confusion during multiple epidemics of influenza at the time. There were numerous cases of post influenza symptoms being falsely diagnosed as pulmonary tuberculosis. In many cases, post influenza would not be diagnosed in time for the lungs to clear up or for tuberculosis bacteria to appear.

Another type of sequelae symptom was caused by a thyroid imbalance. Some cases also showed impaired metabolism of carbohydrates. This would, in turn, lead to increased blood sugar. This could also be brought on by the hypodermic administration of adrenaline. In these cases, the entire endocrine system could be thrown off balance.

The fatigue, nervousness, irritability and rapid heart rate of some cases could be explained in the same way. They were another group of sequelae infections that had been seen in previous epidemics as well.

There were not many cases of gastrointestinal tract symptoms during the initial influenza outbreak. That means that any sequelae symptom dealing with the digestive system are most likely exaggerations of previous problems. One example could be that a patient who suffered a peptic ulcer during his battle with influenza could have a recurrence of the problem. Another example could be a patient who had a biliary tract infection could see a worsening of his condition. It may even lead to colic. There were also very few sequelae cases involving the cardio-vascular or urinary systems. There was little explanation as to why this was. Luckily the common hyperglycemia was mild and did not cause much of a problem like some other symptoms did. There was a sharp increase in these types of cases after the original influenza outbreak. Just as patients started to feel better, they could suffer from these sequelae symptoms.

One interesting and noteworthy sequelae epidemic was called encephalitis lethargica, or "sleeping sickness." It was unclear at the time whether this epidemic was a true post-influenzal infection. However, the time frame in which it occurred is in close relation to influenza. It also followed a near-identical path of spread. Of the five cases observed, three had gotten influenza, and two were free of any previous illness. All five recovered, and the link between influenza and sleeping sickness remained unclear. If sleeping sickness was not directly tied to influenza, it is a strange coincidence.

MORTALITY OF INFLUENZA

One must take into consideration the different forms of influenza while giving a prognosis. It is particularly important to note the possible, and often sudden, changes that can happen in the lungs. The severity and possible negative outcome of influenza can be determined as the following symptoms progress. Cyanosis typically appears early and can indicate the start of a lung infection. It could also be one of the first signs of a worsening case and possible grim outcome. The second sign to watch is body temperature. If a fever developed and fell within a few days, it could point to recovery. However, the prognosis is worse if the fever never breaks, or breaks briefly only to rise again. This could mean that there are lung complications regardless of apparent chest signs. The third sign to watch for is an increased heart rate. The pulse of most influenza patients remained low despite their worsening conditions. If the heart rate did increase, it often pointed to a very bleak outcome. The fourth sign is how the lungs are affected. This was one of the most confusing signs because of its many variables. Say for example that both lower lung lobes become rigid, but the pulse and respiratory rates are good and there is no sign of cyanosis. These cases often made a full recovery. Other cases barely affected the lungs but had a high pulse and cyanosis. These cases were often more severe, possibly fatal. The fifth sign was depression. Remarkably, if a patient remained hopeful and in a good state of mind, their chance of recovery was better than patients who became depressed. This fact remains true regardless of how severe influenza itself was. The Sixth and final sign is the slow and steady increase of respiration rate. Regardless of visible signs, the consistent rise in respiration rate often meant a grim prognosis.

The mortality rate of influenza depended partially on a person's age and health. How quickly one came to the hospital after being infected was another key factor. Take for example the cases of influenza in soldiers. These men were young and healthy. Thanks to these factors, the mortality rate among 153 soldiers was only 10%. Of the 153 soldiers, 66 had lung complications. The civilian cases were a different story. With varying ages and degrees of health, the civilian mortality rate was higher than that of the soldiers. Of 394 civilian patients, the mortality rate was more than 23%. Of the 394 civilians, 237 had lung complications. It could be safely assumed that the older patients' were and the later that they came into the hospital, the higher the mortality rate would be.

Another factor in the mortality rate was the presence of future complications and sequelae infections. Take for example a reported group of 547 patients. Of these patients, 110 had died from complications related to the original influenza virus. 437 patients recovered and were sent home. Before they were discharged, they had been up and walking for 7-10 days. This ensured that they were healthy when they left the hospital. Despite the apparent recovery, many of the patients suffered complications or sequelae infections later. In many of the cases, these patients who thought they had escaped influenza's wrath ended up dying from these later infections. At the time there was no follow-up system in place. This meant that doctors had no way of monitoring the condition of recovered patients. Because of this there was added confusion for doctors trying to diagnose both present cases of influenza and post-influenza infections.

URINE AND BLOOD TESTS

INSPIRED BY THE WORK OF PETER I. ZEEDICK, M. D.

U nlike other epidemics such as scarlet fever and diphtheria, influenza did not attack the kidneys as aggressively. That is, so long as the cases did not develop serious complications. In complicated cases in which toxin and bacteria linked to pneumonia and other complications were involved, there was often swelling in the kidneys. In influenza cases free of complications, the kidneys often escaped unscathed. This is because there was very little swelling of the kidneys in these cases. There had been a few reports that claimed they found higher than normal levels of a protein called albumin in 80% of cases. This is an important blood protein, but high levels can indicate trouble in the kidneys. In contrast to these reports, other claims were made showing anywhere from 4% to 66% of cases with albuminuria. Some reports also claimed that the patients had no signs of pneumonia during the time in which high levels of albuminuria were present. Despite the many observations, it was still agreed that serious, acute kidney swelling was more or less rare.

There had also been past reports of the presence of albumin in the urine. This was most often noticed during the most severe stage of the virus. As this was a common occurrence in other types of infections as well, people paid little attention to it at the time. It was often noted as nothing more than "febrile albuminuria" in many reports. Occasionally, grainy or clear urinary casts were also noticed. Since these things seemed normal for infections, there was little emphasis placed on urinary findings during previous epidemics. It was also found that the inflammation of the kidneys as a separate condition was not prone to follow influenza epidemics.

The following information was collected from 994 urinary samples of 750 patients. The patients were split into two groups. The first group was made up of 517 young men, and the second was a group of 447 men, women and children of various ages. In most cases, only one urine sample was taken from each patient. However, multiple samples were taken from patients who had daily changes or complications. The results were then organized into tables.

The first table shows the urine test results from uncomplicated influenza cases. No patient with an uncomplicated case developed pneumonia. They went on to make full recoveries. Small traces of albuminuria were found in roughly 25% of these patients. There were a few patients who had suffered from previous kidney lesions. High quantities of albuminuria were found in these patients. The presence of this protein didn't typically stick around. It would show up during the worst of the virus and clear up as the patient recovered. More often than not, albuminuria would show up after the patient had a fever for more than two days. In addition, the protein didn't show up in cases lasting

72 hours or less. This pointed to the fact that the patient had to be sick for a certain amount of time before their kidneys were affected. Pneumonia was another factor in the presence of albuminuria. Cases with pneumonia often showed increased levels of the protein. In fact, it was seen around 70% of the time at Magee Hospital. This averages out to show roughly 76% of influenza pneumonia cases had increased levels of the protein. As for the overall epidemic, roughly 40% of all influenza cases had increased albuminuria levels. In addition, 35% of cases with albuminuria also showed casts. However, the number of casts was often low, and casts were often not found in uncomplicated cases.

Red and white blood cells were also seen early in the course of the virus, this could be linked to the nosebleeds and bleeding of the lungs often seen with influenza. The presence of red blood cells in the urine were present in 5% of all influenza cases, and 11% in pneumonia cases. There was never a huge quantity of the blood cells, and there were only a few cases in which the patient's urine became cloudy. Of these, only severe cases had bleeding of the lungs or nose. Some physicians questioned if there could be a link between the presence of blood and albuminuria. However, hemorrhage of the kidneys was never found in influenza cases. The blood cells were most likely an indicator of nephrosis or other toxin complication.

In some cases, there was also the presence of an excess of sugar in the urine. This excess only lasted for short periods of time and never reached dangerous levels. The levels typically stayed within acceptable limits. An interesting note is that diabetic acid and acetone were not found in these cases. The patient's blood sugar levels were kept under control with treatment. It was found that the sugar levels were part of a complication of influenza rather than diabetes or any other ailment. It was thought to be linked to the nervous system and metabolism of carbohydrates. There was one case reported in which the patient suffered nearly complete blindness due to the sugar imbalance. The blood sugar level of the patient rose to around 1% the day they arrived at the hospital. The levels began to drop in the following days until the urine was eventually free of excess sugar. It was unclear how many days the patient's blood sugar was high before they came to the hospital. Though it was near certain that the impairment of vision had begun several weeks prior. A little over two weeks before the patient had started noticing vision problems, they suffered a strong case of influenza. Within a few weeks of arriving at the hospital, the patient recovered and regained their vision. Most patients had fully recovered from influenza before going to the hospital with vision loss or other nervous conditions. Many cases were very similar to those of hyper-thyroidism. This led to the idea that the increased sugar levels were a future complication of influenza that caused the thyroid gland to become hyperactive. This proved to be the most likely explanation.

A related and far more unpleasant sequelae of influenza was furunculosis. This would cause repeated boils to form over the patient's skin. It was obviously painful, and unfortunately, it commonly followed the influenza epidemic. There were often higher than normal levels of sugar in the blood in cases of furunculosis. Despite this, there was no excess sugar, diabetic acid or acetone in the urine. All our blood sugar readings were above the normal, and at times unusually high. The blood sugar levels could be brought under control within a week by getting rid of carbohydrates. In time, this also helped resolve the boils on the skin.

In influenza epidemics of the past, there was little emphasis placed on the specific study of the blood. It was noted that two-thirds of cases maintained normal to low white blood cell counts. The rest showed a gradual increase in white blood cells, mostly after a break in the fevers. Some reports stated that there was no increase in white blood cells during uncomplicated influenza cases and only increased a little in cases with pneumonia. It was also discovered that if the white blood cell numbers began to fall during a case of pneumonia, it usually indicated that the patient was dying. In nearly half of all influenza cases, there was found to be a count of more than 10,000 white blood cells. Some cases even reached as much as 25,000. At the beginning of the illness, the white blood cell count could be as low as 3,000. It then increased as the disease took hold of the patient and fell once more as the fever broke. This curve was important to understanding the changes to the body and blood during influenza. An increase in white blood cells could also indicate a secondary infection. This was one of only a few reported blood results during the epidemic of 1890.

A third of all cases showed a drop in white blood cell numbers. Around 70% of these showed a drop to less than 10,000. This group had more cases of pneumonia than in simple influenza cases. 5% of cases showed a white blood cell count of more than 20,000. It was near guaranteed that these cases would have pneumonia. When pneumonia cases caused by influenza were compared to those of labor pneumonia, it became clear that the two are entirely different. This was part of the confusion for doctors while trying to treat influenza. There were hardly any cases of labor pneumonia in which the white blood cell count was found to be to less than 10,000. This led to the understanding that though the bacteria pneumococcus is present in most forms of pneumonia, it increased in only a low percentage of blood. The toxic factors of influenza are what affect the unusual changes seen in the number of white blood cells.

Most influenza cases without complications should expect normal white blood cell numbers. It is almost certain that any increase in white blood cell numbers indicates a secondary infection. Some cases may see a drop in white blood cells until the fever breaks and the blood cells return to normal levels. In many cases, unidentified sinus infections are to blame for some white blood cell changes after influenza has run its course. In these cases, the drop in white blood cells can be hardly noticeable, or it can be a drastic drop to less than 2,000. The degree to which white blood cell numbers may vary is hardly ever important during uncomplicated cases of influenza, as it varies between cases and typically poses no serious threat to life. It will rebalance itself in time. Since both mild and more severe cases of influenza can show a drop in white blood cells, it can hardly be used to make a prognosis. Unless of course, the case involves pneumonia. While reviewing the results, it is always important to remember that there can easily be human and equipment errors during the counting of blood cells. With such delicate work, pipets and counting chambers should only be trusted if they are certified by the Bureau of Standards.

Specific features of the blood count in cases of pneumonia often varied, but the overall blood picture was consistent across the board. There were typically three different results. The first was an increase in white blood cells, also called leukocytosis. The second was the drop in white blood cell numbers, also called leukopenia. The third was when the number of white blood cells remained steady. Some influenza cases with pneumonia experienced all three.

While the white blood cell numbers fluctuated, the red blood cells were largely unaffected. To better understand this, three groups were observed.

The first group showed an increase of white blood cells during attacks of influenza that led to pneumonia. The group started out with a lowered white blood cell count that then jumped to a count of between 10,000 and 15,000 as soon as the pneumonia set in. The white blood cells hardly ever exceeded a count of 20,000. As the patients recovered, their white blood cell count returned to normal. On occasion, these patients would suffer a secondary lung complication, in which case the white blood cell count would rise again. These cases were often fatal. Another possibility is that the white blood cell numbers would drop after the initial rise in number. The longer the cell count remained high before dropping, the more serious the case could become once the number dropped.

The second group consisted of patients whose white blood cell count remained low throughout the course of influenza. These cases were common. This is a cardinal point—in fact, one of the most striking clinical features of the epidemic. A drop to between 4,000 and 5,000 was typically safe. A drop to 3,000 or less could prove to be very serious and potentially indicate a grim outcome. In cases with pneumonia, the patient often died when the white blood cell count fell to around 2,000. In the cases where the patient did recover, the cell count was able to balance itself to a rather normal number.

The third group showed a split between high white blood cell counts and a low count. There was a fair number of pneumonia cases within this group. In these cases, a drop in white blood cell numbers after a period of stabilizing is often a bad sign. A rise in white blood cells, on the other hand, could be a good thing. In these cases, there was often a sudden rise in white blood cells to around 20,000 later in the illness. The rise would often continue until the end of the illness and often meant that the patient was on their way to recovering.

TREATING INFLUENZA

INSPIRED BY THE WORK OF W. W. G. MACLACHLAN, M. D.

At the time of previous influenza epidemics, there was no clear treatment. Symptoms could be managed in a clinical setting, but there was no one cure for the virus itself. The attack of these influenza outbreaks was a wake-up call to humanity, and it brought with it a healthy dose of humility. It was clear that more research had to be done in order to understand the virus. In doing so, the medical community might also be able to prepare for future disease outbreaks. With such short bursts of influenza outbreaks and a shortage of physicians, it was hard for much study to be done. The research that was completed was still of value. Any new information on the disease was helpful, even if it was only a little information.

The treatment of influenza was broken into three groups. These groups were acute influenza, pneumonia, and other complications. No specific drug was thoroughly proven to be effective, but there were several in use to treat acute influenza. These included alkalies, antipyretics, quinine, salicylates, and the sedatives. Each drug had a number of followers who claimed that it was the best treatment, though there was little agreement between groups. One agreement across the board was that the use of coal tar was not advisable. Other methods of treatment date back to the 16th century. These included sweating out the virus aided by the use of diaphoretics, getting enough fresh air, restricting one's diet, and leaving mild cases to be healed in time. Some of these old, simple remedies are still of value today.

Pneumonia was a big factor in the mortality rate of influenza. Serum and blood therapy was sometimes used to treat pneumonia caused by influenza. This method included using the blood of recovering patients. Physicians would transfer blood or serum from recovering patients to sick patients in the hope that it would help the sick person fight off the infection. The treatment had been proven useful in previous outbreaks such as those of scarlet fever. This was left as an emergency treatment option.

Another complication of influenza was that of the nervous system. These complications often came after the patient had apparently recovered from the virus. In some cases, these complications included temporary vision loss or impairment. Only symptom relief methods such as removing carbohydrates were available. These efforts still proved beneficial in aiding the recovery of these patients. Since the outbreak of 1890, there have been very few cases of nervous system complications due to influenza.

Vaccines were another treatment method that came later in the development of influenza treatments. Vaccines would go on to become the number one weapon against influenza and are still used to this day. In the early days of vaccine research, having accurate and honest clinical reports were of utmost importance. Any miscalculation or false information could lead to failure of treatment. More importantly, it could be dangerous for the patients.

Regardless of if the case was mild or severe, there was one very important part of the influenza treatment: rest. Going to bed early and remaining well-rested throughout the duration of the virus was vital to recovery. Most patients would go to bed willingly. However, there were cases in which a patient refused to rest. They would try to push through any discomfort. This stubbornness might increase the patient's chance of developing serious pneumonia. Even if the case of influenza seems mild, the patient should stay in bed until their fever breaks and all other signs return to normal. A hot bath followed by hot drinks with lemon could also provide much relief to patients. This is good advice even today. We now know how important it is to rest when sick, and we are all familiar with how comforting a warm bath or hot tea with lemon can be when sick.

A good nurse would keep the patient covered and warm and give the patient plenty of water. A cold compress to the head can be beneficial, but cold sponging is not often recommended. The patient should not be allowed to rise for any reason. The room temperature should be watched carefully, and the patient should be allowed fresh air so long as the weather was warm. The patient may lose their appetite early in the illness, but this is normal and should not be of much concern. Soft foods and drinks can be given during this time until the patient has more of an appetite. It was found that meat broths could add to inflammation of the kidneys and should therefore be avoided until the patient is in recovery.

These "soft" treatments were not the only methods used. Some treatment methods worked in certain cases, but they could also be potentially dangerous. For example, quinine sulfate was used until it was found to cause deafness. Another drug used was acetylsalicylic acid. This was used to treat bad headaches. The effects of this drug were also questionable. In addition to these, a salt called sodium bicarbonate was added to the patients' water to increase urine flow and flush out the kidneys. A calomel purge and saline, castor oil, and magnesium sulfate were other methods used to help treat influenza once the average severity of all cases dropped.

The respiratory symptoms were the most concerning of influenza symptoms. Because of this, treatment for these symptoms was of utmost importance. Ammonium chloride was typically prescribed to help treat coughs. It helped chronic cases the most. Mucus loosening terpin with heroin, sleep-inducing codeine and the occasional dose of morphine were given regularly to help symptoms. Benzoin infused steam followed, spraying the throat with medicated liquid petroleum was also said to give some relief. giving some relief. Some treatments, including those involving inhalers, were warned against in cases complicated by pneumonia. At the start of the epidemic, even whisky was prescribed in most cases. It was thought to have sedative effects. In time the value of whisky became questionable. We now know that several of these treatments are more than questionable. Whiskey for example, like all alcohol, is now known to suppress the immune system and can lead to a longer recovery time.

PNEUMONIA

Pneumonia often followed the original influenza infection. This pneumonia was difficult to diagnose in its early stages, as there was quite a lot of overlap between the initial influenza infection and the subsequent bacterial one. It was not uncommon for seemingly mild cases of influenza to develop into life-threatening cases of pneumonia. The previously described treatments were given to patients up to the point in which pneumonia was found. From here, the treatment methods changed. This is because of the further complications brought on by pneumonia, and the potential risk of some previous treatments at this stage of the virus.

Dedicated nurses who looked after the patient and helped the patient conserve their energy were still of great value. So was the fact that the patient should be kept warm and covered and given plentiful water and fresh air. The patient should be kept on a light diet. The specific diet depends on the severity of the case. As a good rule of thumb, it was always safer to limit the patient to a fluid diet while the pneumonia was still present. Once the pneumonia had cleared up, the patient's diet could be increased rather quickly.

Castor oil was recommended to help the patient have easier bowel movements. It was recommended to use castor oil every other day, or as the patient needed it. There was often less abdominal distention during cases of influenza pneumonia that there was with lobar pneumonia. Plain soap with turpentine was often injected into the rectum to help ease cases of abdominal distention. This method provided good results. Most importantly, the patient needed to rest. Morphine could help the patient sleep comfortably when needed.

In early epidemics, it was not possible to separate the pneumonia cases from the rest of the influenza cases. This was in part due to the overwhelming number of patients, and the strain placed on doctors and nurses. However, in future epidemics, a system of separation would be more likely. This would be of great benefit to physicians as well as the patients. It was not uncommon for patients to develop pneumonia from the patient next to them. This is why it was vital to separate the pneumonia patients and other patients as much as possible. It was also important to separate patients within the same group as much as possible. This is because a recovering patient could be re-infected by a sick patient next to them. In a number of hospitals, the separation was made possible with ward sheets. These sheets would stretch between beds to prevent any cross-contamination of sick patients. This was perhaps the easiest way of providing a separation between patients.

Quinine, salicylates, and salol did not seem to help after the start of pneumonia. At the time of this realization, these drugs were no longer used. Digitalis drugs dissolved in alcohol were regularly used as a replacement. This too was given up on by the middle of the epidemic.

In cases of uncomplicated pneumonia, the heart was not clearly involved. A slow, steady pulse was typical, and it did not need the use of drugs. The respiratory system was the main concern. Remedies included caffeine, salicylate, and sodium benzoate. These appeared to be of great value to patients. This is because these are respiratory stimulants. They also helped increase urine production, supposedly helping the kidneys. These were given often. In addition, atropine was given if fluid retention or swelling were noticed. This was not always useful, though it was believed to save a few lives in severe cases.

After many failed attempts, the creation of a useful immune serum was a great achievement for the medical community. With this in mind, it is important to remember the differences between influenza pneumonia and labor pneumonia, as the serum could affect them differently. It was also exceptionally hard to get the valuable anti-pneu-mococci immune serum during the epidemic. This meant that it could not be used in treatment like people hoped it would be. The army had roughly half a dozen bottles available, but that was it. After this was used, there was no more available. A similar serum was the anti-pneumococci chicken serum. It had a small trial but proved to be highly beneficial. Though this serum was also largely unavailable for widespread use, it was a start. These serums paved the way for future treatments.

The severity of pneumonia caused by influenza and the apparent helplessness of doctors to do anything about it was startling. For further testing, there was a study done on a group of roughly 100 Student Army Training Corps soldiers from Pittsburgh University. Several important things were found within the first week. First was the incredibly high mortality rate of severe cases of influenza pneumonia. At the time, most cases of pneumonia were severe. This is certainly a contributing factor to the overall mortality rate. The second interesting discovery was that the cases varied widely. All the soldiers had come from the same place. Despite sharing a common environment, each soldier had a different level of severity with influenza. This range of severity was puzzling, but it eventually led to a better understanding of how to treat the disease.

A hypothesis was formed that patients recovering from mild cases developed higher immunity to the virus than those suffering more severe cases. This led to the theory that this immunity might be able to be transferred to other patients. This came from the idea that immune bodies could be found in the blood if mild cases did in fact show greater immunity build up. In theory, this immunity to rich blood could be transferred from a recovering patient to a patient sick with a more severe case of influenza. When this method was eventually tested, the outcomes were remarkably favorable. Whole blood was used in order to simplify and speed up the process. Similar types of blood therapy are still being used in medicine today.

The use of blood or the immune serum from recovering patients proved extremely beneficial to pneumonia patients. There were several reports made on the effectiveness of this method of treatment. One report noted 30 recoveries out of 37 and only one death. Another report showed only 6 deaths out of 151 cases. This was a dramatic improvement in the mortality rate. It was irrefutable proof that this method worked.

To review, both serum and whole blood can be used in the treatment of influenza. This is particularly of use for severe cases or cases involving pneumonia. Some groups believe that whole blood has stronger bacterial properties and immunity benefits than serum or plasma. That being said, there are no cons of using serum. Either way, the therapy has proven beneficial. The use of whole blood is faster, but it must be noted that there is a factor that the blood will clump together. When introducing new blood, it is vital to properly calculate and account for this reaction. This practice also carries the risk of donor deaths. Obviously, military and hospital settings are well regulated. In these settings, donors do not die from the blood transfer. This is because, in clinical settings, the amount of whole blood given was typically between 50 cc. and 75 cc. If treated early, 50 cc. of blood can do just as much good as 100 cc. of blood. Transfusions in the clinical setting never exceeded the safety limit of 100 cc. However, the practice had also been picked up by the civilian practice. This is when problems started to arise. In some cases there were reports of civilian practices giving up to 500 cc. of whole blood. This is way above the safe amount. The disregard of clinical standards led to multiple complications and deaths.

There were several other differences between the military and civilian sectors. Soldiers were often more than willing to give blood. Their job, after all, is to serve and protect the country. As they were happy to donate blood, there was never any shortage of military donors. It proved a little more difficult to get the civilian population to willingly donate blood. People were obviously ready and willing to donate blood to save a friend or family member, but only a few friends and family cases. People were less likely to be willing to donate blood for a stranger. This meant that it was hard to find civilian donors. This made it much harder to get enough blood to treat all the cases. The process of taking blood does not have to be a scary or difficult surgical process. With the use of a syringe, the process is simple and near painless. Regardless of advancements, it was still hard for physicians to find enough donors for the many cases needing blood.

This was made more difficult by the pressure of time. The sooner pneumonia is recognized, the better the chance of recovery. By this time physicians were fairly confident that lung lesions were present if the patient's fever remained high for more than four days. Later stages of pneumonia did not react as well to the blood transfusion. This is because the serum only works well in the initial stages of influenza. There were very few deep pneumonia cases that recovered. Unfortunately, there is no treatment for cases of this intense severity.

Even after successful treatment, the white blood cell count remained relatively unchanged. This was a rather surprising result when considering the group as a whole. There were other results in which the outcomes of the injections were positive, and the number of white blood cells increased. Cases in which the patient's white blood cell count was below 10,000 had the best results. This could mean that the original influenza virus has the biggest impact, and secondary infections have less of a role. That is why early treatment is vital.

Based on the results, it is clear that blood, or immune serum, is the best treatment when used early on in the influenza infection. For that reason, it was advised to continue the use of this method unless a better treatment was found. It was also advised to start the use of this treatment as early as possible during future epidemics.

Records were kept of the ward charts of studies following patients who developed pneumonia after the original influenza virus. The charts show the effects of using the immunity serum in these pneumonic cases. The charts highlighted in this section are those of the patients who recovered. The charts of those who unfortunately passed away showed nothing of great value other than the slim chance that these patients had after treatment. From the charts, several key results were shown. The following are some such results.

(1) In most cases, the fever broke after the patient received the injection.

(2) Occasional chills after the injections showed little valuable or noteworthy results.

(3) After the injection, there is typically little to no change in white blood cell counts. It was also shown that cases with counts of 10,000 or less had the best results after the injection.

(4) In many cases the injection was not able to be given until later in the course of the virus. This was obviously not ideal. For better results, the injections should have been given much sooner.

(5) Several charts show that only one injection of 50 cc. is all that's necessary if it is given early. There was little added benefit to giving more than 50 cc. to a patient, and it was never advised to give more than 100 cc. for any reason.

(6) Pneumonia typically starts showing signs after a spike in body temperature after influenza has run its course. Information about pneumonia and when it started is not shown in the charts. This is because it was recorded in daily notes instead.

Complications

Most complications began after the patient had seemingly recovered from the influenza virus. The exception to this was lung complications which could arise during the initial virus or directly after the initial influenza. Many different future complications arose. However, connecting all future ailments to past epidemics was warned against. The various complications that were shown and the treatments for them are not discussed in great detail. Only the main points will be highlighted.

Pneumonia is closely associated with influenza. It is in fact the main complication of the disease. Non-resolution and fibrosis are the most important end results of pneumonia. Unfortunately, at the time, there were not many useful treatments for this complication. The main treatment attempt was good nursing and providing as many nutrients as possible. Maintaining hygienic conditions was also valued during attempted treatment. Sponging the patient with warm water provided some relief to the patient. It helped control excess sweating. Some drugs were also used but were only valuable in a few cases. Thoughtful and careful vaccine therapy was also discussed as a possible treatment if used early. Pneumonia often lasted several weeks, and the chances of recovery were slim.

Pus was not found as often as one would imagine between the lung and the inner chest wall. With such a lack of success in the healing of the lungs after pneumonia, the little amount of pus was surprising. Needles were used to explore any case that the healing process was taking longer than expected. This allowed physicians to feel the condition of the chest and identify if there was pus present. Surgery is the typical treatment for any excess of pus. There were a few new drainage techniques in question, though they had not been thoroughly tested. Most cases in which the pus was discovered and treated did well.

Chest pain was another complication complaint. Pain and discharge in the pleura section of the chest was reported several times. Few cases were found with a large amount of discharge. The signs may not indicate a puncture in the pleura even if one was present. These cases often had bad results. When it was found to be present, the fluid was aspirated. When this was done, the end results were good. After the aspiration of the fluid was done, it hardly ever needed to be repeated. There was only one reported case of a repeated aspiration.

Chronic bronchitis was another complication some-times reported. Some patients also reported having difficulty breathing with this complication. This was most often associated with some form of lung fibrosis. It was also likely associated with the small bronchioles. There was a variation of matter being coughed up in these cases. Some cases had a lot of coughed up matter, and others had very little. Some cases also had mucus and pus present in the matter. The best treatment for this was rest and nutrients. It was recommended that the patient stays in bed and gets as rich of a diet as possible to help them build strength. In the first cases, rest was not deemed essential. That is because these cases often do not show a fever. However, as time passed, it became apparent that rest was necessary to the recovery of these patients. At times, atropine and heroin were used and shown to be of some value. Physicians were often surprised that this specific complication was not more common.

Phlebitis, or inflammation of the veins, was also seen in some cases. It typically affected the femoral vein, one of the larger veins in the leg. This was just as common with the influenza virus as it was for typhoid fever. Luckily, the influenza cases showed much better results than those of typhoid fever. There was only one reported, a severe case that affected the patient's leg. The usual treatment was simply rest and elevation of the affected limb. If the patient was in pain during the most severe stage, ice could be carefully applied. It is important that the limb is rested for several weeks to ensure a full recovery.

Acute sinus infection was another fairly common complication. This could happen while the original influenza illness was still in effect. Though, it was more commonly seen after the initial infection. Some cases didn't develop until weeks after the patient had recovered from influenza. The most vulnerable part of the sinuses. This is where most infections were located. There were also a good number of infections in the frontal sinuses. This second type of infection usually began during or immediately after the original influenza virus. Most of the infections were temporary and cleared up with localized treatment. In fact, cold applications were often the only necessary treatment for frontal sinus infections. Surgery was sometimes necessary for more serious, chronic infections. The surgery usually proved to be an effective treatment. Given the number of influenza patients, ear infections were not as common. If necessary, the eardrum was punctured and drained. At the time, this was an effective treatment for severe ear infections.

There were a handful of meningitis cases reported to be associated with influenza pneumonia cases. In these cases, a culture of the pneumococcus was made from the spinal fluid. From here, it was recommended that an anti-pneumo-coccus serum was injected into the spinal column. The serum helped several cases recover if given early in the infection.

Cases of vision impairment or loss were seen on occasion after the epidemic of 1890. Optic swelling, inflamed peripheral nerves, and excess sugar in the urine were often seen in these cases. There were also a few cases in which there was an excess of sugar in the urine but no clear eye symptoms. These cases may still be tied to the nervous system complications that caused the eye issues. Rest and the flushing of toxins were the primary treatment. Calomel was used to help empty the gastrointestinal tract, followed by several days of saline given in the morning. Hot packs were sometimes used for up to two weeks to ease symptoms. Sugar, bread and some vegetables were removed from the patient's diet, and they were instructed to drink as much water as possible. With this treatment, the excess sugar in the urine dissipated within roughly three days.

The vision slowly improved, but it could take up to five weeks to return to normal. The patient was kept in bed for three weeks after arriving at the hospital. The patients without eye issues required very little treatment. It didn't take anything more than a carbohydrate-free diet to treat these cases and remove the excess sugar from their system. A test was done to see how a non-restricted diet would affect the patients. The cases cleared up after a few days despite the sugar in their diet. These cases were not given hot packs, yet ease of bowel movements remained present. The cases were recognized by regular examinations of the urine and were not linked to diabetes mellitus.

PREVENTION OF INFLUENZA

INSPIRED BY THE WORK OF SAMUEL R. HAYTHORN, M. D.

In regard to vaccination, influenza has proven one of the most elusive biological opponents to be handled by preventive medication. This led to substantial divisiveness and the formation of advocacy and opponent groups of this specific type of prevention. In order to better understand this, it would be reasonable to return to the more fundamental processes by which vaccines work to provide more information on this matter.

This first-time vaccine word was incorporated into the English language was in 1796, when it was discovered that virus taken from cowpox pustules provided immunity against the smallpox virus, which is closely related in lineage. Eventually, the term came to mean all forms of inoculation that later provide immunity to a pathogen (i.e., a virus or bacteria). Methods of producing vaccine varied: sometimes the virus is grown in an animal that cannot contract the illness, sometimes viruses are taken apart so that only the benign parts are given to the individual, a term known as attenuation, and in many bacterial cases, the organism is often killed and the vaccine created from the remains. Vaccines are used to create immunity and prevent infection, whereas a different kind of treatment, named sera, is used for active treatment of illness by using immune components created by the live animals growing the virus to fight it inside the patient. The smallpox vaccine was the first of its kind and proved to completely eradicate the disease. Rabies is another example in which vaccination had proven to largely to prevent disease. The killed bacteria type of vaccine emerged in 1896, brought about by Sir Almroth Wright, and had proven to control a host of other diseases (typhoid, dysentery, etc.).

Bacterial vaccination had a benefit of simple production using basic lab equipment, where the bacteria is grown, killed using various methods, and put into a solution that is used later for injection. These usually take multiple doses to create immunity. More recently, a suspension created by Fennel and Peterson in oil allowed for the dose to increase without creating harm, reducing the amount of doses to one (termed lipovaccines). The typhoid vaccine started using this approach shortly after invention. Another method, known as sensitization, involved putting the bacterial vaccines on the same growth plate as serum taken from animals that had been immunized. This additionally increased the effectiveness of these vaccines. There was some attempts to use live bacteria using this method, but this is rarely used because live bacteria increases the chance that the vaccine could still be harmful.

Vaccines usually produce a mild fever and soreness around the injection site, starting about 12 hours after injection and lasting as long as 48 hours. This is part of the body's overall immune response to the new pathogen as it creates memory cells designed to identify it in the future. The body's immune system can effectively recognize the new pathogen a few days after administration of the vaccine. Several scientists show that this is caused by specific substances that act on the bacteria and allow it to be identified by the immune cells of the body. In animals, it has been proven that this response can be heightened to the point where a normally fatal dose of bacteria will no longer have the same effect. Interestingly, if bacteria have similar components from closely related members of its family, vaccination will provide some protection against these as well.

The most successful bacterial vaccine developed to this point had been for typhoid fever, which ravaged the United States Army during the Spanish War, causing over 20,000 men to fall ill in U.S. camps and 1580 deaths. When another war occurred in the summer of 1911, and the vaccine had been provided to 12,801 men in infantry in San Antonio, Texas, there were only two cases and no fatalities. The year after this, typhoid vaccination became compulsory in the United States Army. The only outbreak of typhoid that occurred between then and 1918 was an 18-case burst at Camp Greene, Charlotte, N.C, of which six of the men had not completed the immunization process. Indeed, vaccination had become a prominent member in preventive medicine during this time.

VACCINATION AGAINST INFLUENZA

The difficulty of preparing a vaccine for influenza started with the elusiveness of its causative organism. To this point, there had been no consensus on the organism that caused this illness, with the most promising idea being Pfeiffer bacillus (also known as B. influenzae), to which no relationship had been conclusively demonstrated.

Experiments that were started to prove the connection between this bacteria and influenza yielded confusing results. At first, in a small experiment using 16 men receiving the B. Pfeiffer vaccine, followed by secretions and blood from typical influenza cases, resulted in no cases of influenza. However, a similar experiment was performed in San Francisco using a vaccine of different bacteria, also produced the same results. This left the question as to the cause of influenza still remaining.

Those who were not convinced of B. Pfeiffer's connection to influenza posed the idea that its presence in cases of influenza were a result of secondary invasion, something that can occur when viruses infect the body. This was also supported by the fact that the bacteria was not always found in all cases of this illness, as well as the fact that inoculation with pure live strains of the bacteria does not always produce disease, either in man or animals. Those that believed its connection cited the high rate of presence in respiratory secretions of patients suffering from influenza, its predilection for the respiratory tract, and that transfer of influenza fails from man to man when Pfeiffer bacilli are used. They also cited the fact that it is difficult to retrieve respiratory cultures, and that when deceased influenza patients were autopsied and their lungs cultured, the rate of the bacteria increased. Some scientists also argued that a change in morphology by the bacteria could make identification more difficult. Indeed, it was apparent that the argument against B. Pfeiffer would lose weight when the difficulty of respiratory secretions was considered.

Due to this dispute and the relative lack of any other leading causative organism. At the start of the 1918 epidemic, Pfeiffer bacillus was generally thought to be the cause. It was only later realized that most influenza deaths were due to complicating pneumonias that this information came into play. Using this information, attempts were then begun to create a specific vaccine against this organism.

Vaccines against infectious diseases are commonly made from parts of the causative organism that will activate the immune system to create a memory of said organism. The idea is that the unique parts of this organism will create a signature that will be recognized by the immune system specifically as being the infectious organism without causing a reaction to other kinds of material that look similar. This was the concept used when the Pfeiffer vaccine creation was undertaken to prevent infection.

Several Pfeiffer vaccines had been tried in treatment, but this was still a relatively new undertaking at this time. Many companies had influenza vaccines already on the market for treatment, most of which contained Pfeiffer bacteria. There were two cases of sinus infection that were treated with Pfeiffer vaccines, one of which the patient improved rapidly and one where there was no change. On investigation of several other vaccines, they were found to have mixed components. Some work had been completed by Flexner and Wolstein using serum prepared from Pfeiffer bacillus, which was able to cure monkeys of influenza meningitis. However, this treatment did not have effect on human subjects.

The first-time pure Pfeiffer vaccines were used to prevent influenza were by Leary and Rosenau. Leary used his vaccine in Boston both for influenza treatment and prevention, with the preventive vaccine being given to medical students and nurses. It seemed initially promising; however, follow-up results did not prevail along hopeful lines. Barnes was able to test his vaccine in an institution near Woonsocket, after three patients were diagnosed with influenza. The vaccine was given to 172 employees and patients over 3 days following the diagnosis of the most recent patient. Close to 35 people had contracted the illness before all three doses were administered, for which they were removed from the statistical analysis. When the results were calculated, the vaccine failed to show any benefit in preventing or treating any cases during this outbreak. Hinton and Kane used the Leary vaccine at the Monson State Hospital in the most complete and scientifically rigorous experiment on a population of 979 inmates, and conclusively showed that the vaccine failed to protect individuals against the illness.

Successive attempts to prove this vaccine as effective were not as well controlled, and in actuality, promoted the failure of the vaccine. Taunton State Hospital and Gardner State Colony were two studies that both had over 800 participants but was performed after the peak of the epidemic had passed. The Massachusetts School for Feeble-Minded had another large-scale study of 457 inmates but had issues with selection of participants. Wrentham State School was both undertaken after the peak and comments that the vaccinated were not as ill as the unvaccinated. Medfield State Hospital was also undertaking their study after the peak. North Hampton State Hospital failed to show any difference between vaccine and control groups. Westerborough State Hospital saw a slight increase in deaths in the vaccinated group.

A report later drawn up that analyzed the studies performed on over 6,000 vaccinated patients reported that the vaccine did not prevent or treat influenza, nor did it cause any harm. This resulted in the definitive conclusion of the trials performed in Massachusetts.

A second Pfeiffer bacilli vaccine, using bacteria isolated from cases of influenza during this pandemic, was being developed for use at the Chelsea Naval Hospital in Pelham Bay. This study was carried out on an isolated group of officers that were practically free of influenza. This experiment began on September 30, using the same protocol of 3 doses given 24 hours apart. A total of 565 men were full vaccinated to serve as the experimental group, who were then transferred about the Naval service to various locations. The influenza rate of both the control and experimental groups were tracked over the next 14 days. At the conclusion of the experiment, the results failed to show any protective qualities of the experimental solution.

The New York City Board of Health also sponsored vaccine production during this time, who's method was overseen by W.H. Parke. These vaccines contained 17 different strains of Pfeiffer bacteria, isolated from influenza cases during the pandemic. The vaccination schedule was also altered, so that there were 3 doses given at seven-day intervals. However, there was no obtainable data that emerged from this experiment.

Haythorn also, at the request of the city of Pittsburgh, followed Parke's method of preparing the vaccine to manu-facture large quantities to be distributed. This work began at Singer Memorial Laboratory, using 13 different strains of Pfeiffer bacilli, obtained by autopsy and fresh culture. The techniques used by W.H. Parke were adhered to, with only slight variation as the performing scientists saw fit to produce more dependable results. The final sample was tested on mice and guinea pigs to assure it would not be toxic to human subjects. The first 5 liters of vaccine were turned over to the Red Cross one week later, on October 31. However, it was on day 5 that an order was passed down to discontinue production. This vaccine became mixed into others during distribution, so it was not possible to tell its effect. However, Haythorn and his colleagues took the remaining bacteria and tested it on animal models, namely mice and guinea pigs. It was here that it was found that they could not find enough of a dose to be lethal to animals: thus, they were unable to determine a starting point for the protective effect of the vaccine. The scientists hypothesized that keeping the bacteria in lab culture for so long could have reduced its potency, but nevertheless, concluded that the Pfeiffer vaccine was ultimately a failure in its current form.

INFLUENZA PREVENTIVE MEASURES

One of the most concerning aspects of the 1918 influenza pandemic was the rate at which it spread. The distance between the first case in Boston and the first in San Francisco was less than two months, with the peaks in each city about one month apart. No habitable part of the world was unaffected by the illness. Societal factors contributed to the spread as well; due to the war, most were living in close quarters to other individuals, and thousands of men were housed in army camps. Also, the distribution of wartime materials or rebuilding war-afflicted countries brought many people from largely different areas into the same commune. Since resources were scarce, levels of fatigue and nervousness were at a level higher than normal. These types of social changes likely both increased exposure to the illness and decreased the body's ability to respond to its inhabitance. It was the first wave that contributed to the major amount of mortality as well, which happened so acutely that no method of prevention or treatment could rightly be proven or disproven at the end of such efforts.

In December 1918, the American Public Health Association held a meeting in Chicago, with the express purpose of categorizing and documenting the extent and methods of prevention of the outbreak. They concluded few things at the end of this meeting, that the disease was probably caused by some micro-organism or virus not yet known, and spread via the noses and mouths of infected persons, that there was no known laboratory methods to decipher it from other types of respiratory illness, that it was presently unknown when a patient was no longer infective, and that most deaths were due to secondary infection and pneumonia resulting from a different bacteria. Indeed, the little amount of information posed a grim scenario.

The few conclusions that the APHA decided to pursue in order to limit the recurrence of the illness were to stop the spread of the illness. Secondary, it would be important to determine how to increase immunity of persons exposed to infection. Finally, the goal would be to increase the natural resistance of persons to disease. The methods of these three goals will be taken into further deliberation in the passages below.

QUARANTINE TO STOP THE SPREAD

The first method for stopping the spread of the illness involved a strict quarantine for affected persons. This was advocated by many both in the field and the public. The distribution of spread made it apparent that the disease spread most rapidly when people were congregated in large groups. This kind of quarantine was appealing for both limiting the spread and reducing exposure of the patient to the kinds of bacteria that result in a second infection and are the large cause of death in influenza patients. From a standpoint of epidemiology, this made sense.

Several issues were posed against quarantine during the meeting, as to why it was not logically feasible in this scenario. The first of these were the lack of a proper diagnosing method, especially in the early stages when the patient is infective. This could possibly have led to large amounts of unjust quarantines and wasted resources, and a delay in diagnosis that could render quarantining the patient basically ineffective, for their part in the spread will have already been done. Also, the infective capability of the illness would have required quarantine of all close contacts of patients to be effective, which, when drawn out, would rapidly become such a substantial amount of the population that the economy would be brought to a halt. Additionally, if the infected patient was able to transmit before they became symptomatic, which was starting to become known at that time due to the failure to contain the disease by removing symptomatic soldiers from their barracks, then quarantine at that point, even if caught at the earliest symptom, would be futile as a sole means of prevention.

A secondary, less rigid isolation method, termed the Cubicle System, was also proposed. This consisted of dividing rooms into small compartments so that each person is separated by suspended sheets. Camp Grant showed some positive results using this method. This came with the additional requirement that anyone entering or leaving the cubicle would be forced to wear a mask. This had been demonstrated previously at the Pasteur Institute of Paris, and in control of diphtheria, measles, and scarlet fever. Combining this method with good hygiene and hand washing was determined worthy of trial.

USE OF THE FACE MASK

I t was undetermined at this point whether wearing a mask over the mouth had any benefit during the epidemic. There had been prior history of using masks to prevent other diseases up to this point. Masks were shown in 1917 to reduce the percentage of diphtheria carriers among nurses in the Durand Hospital of Infectious Disease almost 75%. It was this type of information that led to the recommendation that physicians use masks when coming into contact with all types of respiratory diseases. The study done at Camp Grant, which utilized masks, showed favorable outcomes. This became a popular recommendation against the influenza epidemic.

Experiments to determine the efficacy of masks generally were done by spraying bacteria over a lab plate covered by a gauze. Conversely, it was also tested by having a person wear a mask and cough over a plate, to determine if they reduced transmission. These were fairly reliable laboratory experiments, and they determined that the efficacy of the mask was directly related to the fineness of the mesh and the number of layers used.

Drs. Doust and Lyon came up with an additional layer of experiments that determined the distance that droplets can carry under various life circumstances. Their results found that ordinary speech can carry infected material roughly 4 feet, and that during coughing it can travel as far as ten. They tested this hypothesis with medium mesh gauze between two and ten layers thick and determined that coughing did not prevent the spread of infectious material. However, when a butter cloth mask was used, it was much more efficient. These tests were furthered by Haller and Colwell, who concluded that a five-layer mask made of 24x20 mesh protected growth onto a plate. This was replicated several times, with the addition of a wire frame to the masks that allowed it to keep dry, which all scientists agreed improved its effectiveness.

When information on the efficacy of masks was discussed, most agreed that it was a helpful intervention, although not fully preventive. There were cases where patients who wore masks diligently still contracted the disease, but when these numbers were measured against individuals not wearing masks, the number was substantially lower. The best case for masks came from the parallels between San Francisco and Los Angeles during the epidemic. San Francisco started using masks universally before Los Angeles employed the same strategy and saw a sharper decline in the rate of cases. When Los Angeles instituted a mask-wearing policy, they saw a similar rate of decline. It was agreed at the conclusion that masks were useful in combating influenza, even if the effectiveness was at times overstated.

GENERAL CLOSING ORDERS

Most large gatherings in cities were prohibited during this time. Intriguingly, New York did not follow suit in closing large public gatherings and had a death rate lower than several other large cities. These numbers, however, were not specifically following people who attended gatherings vs. those who did not.

It was agreed upon that unnecessary public gatherings were inadvisable and had been the policy during any epidemic. It was interesting to note that, even in well-ventilated areas, overcrowding was a more important issue that needed to be prevented. There was some resistance that closing public meeting spaces could incite panic and only delay the epidemic, but these were not substantiated.

Most places were initially resistant to closing public schools, due to the backlash with anxious parents. It was argued that children were relatively unaffected by the illness, and that close monitoring of the children could provide adequate coverage. In New York, it was argued that children were far better off in school with access to medical care, then cordoned off at home in potentially unsuitable environments. On the converse side, the arguments against keeping schools open was threefold: it was undetermined to what extent the illness could be carried by children and keeping them open could potentiate the spread, it was unjust to force kids from cleaner homes into schools with children from unclean homes, and the monitoring of symptoms in children was useless, since the greatest period of infectivity arose before symptoms occur. It was clear that these kind of considerations should be made on a case-by-case basis for each school.

Public dances were unquestionably prohibited during the epidemic. Interestingly, these people were somewhat even more susceptible, as it was hypothesized that alternate overheating and rapid cooling of the body led to decreased resistance.

Because public eating places could not be altogether closed due to their necessity, cautions were put in place to limit the spread as much as possible. People were warned against using these forums as areas for congregation and entertainment. It was also expected that the Board of Health and restaurants take extra precautions to sterilize their dishware and eating spaces, as well as daily inspection of employees, to prevent spread. Soda fountains were determined to be a large source of spread, and recommendation for closure was given unless they could be held to the absolute highest standards. Establishments were encouraged to use paper dishes and glasses, scalding all reusable utensils, and use exceptional cleanliness when preparing food, as hand-to-mouth spread was just as quick as respiratory spread.

It was evident at this time that business must continue, and traffic was an essential component to that. This was a concern during this time, as public transport in larger cities is generally loaded to capacity for several hours throughout the day. This was first approached in the city of Pittsburgh by warnings placed in public transit against coughing, spitting, and sneezing. These warnings also instructed people to go home if the fell ill. Not long after, a second order was placed to raise all windows six inches, and to turn off the heat in public transport vehicles, in order to improve ventilation. This was not an effective method, however, as cold days and rain led to decreased compliance. The cold also led to more people crowding into warmer areas of the vehicles, which very well could have increased transmission.

In New York, public transportation was approached with a "stagger-hour" system, which changed working hours of businesses so that the rush traffic would not be as severe during the beginning and end hours of the day. This would decrease the amount of people the vehicles carried per hour.

After all the methods were analyzed, it seemed that the most effective measures for decreasing spread were the warning signs, the stagger-hour system, and general guidance to avoid public transport as much as possible. These were deemed effective enough to have in place for the next epidemic.

ANTI-SPITTING ORDINANCES

All public transport had signs that warned against spitting, under penalty of fine and imprisonment. These ordinances were rarely followed during normal times. It was certainly an unsightly act from a hygienic standpoint but was rarely enforced as a punishable act. It was recommended that these be enforced, as well as teaching the dangers of spreading disease through spitting to children, not just for influenza, but for prevention of the spread of other transmissible diseases.

The interesting demographic finding in influenza was that it tended to be the best trained, most healthful individuals who suffered the most. This was namely expressed by the amount of military personnel afflicted with hit. It seemed that the intense respiratory effort that came from physical training could have led to increased transmission. Thus, it was reasonable at this time to suggest that people should get more rest and healthy food, to enjoy more relaxation than strenuous exercise, to wear warmer clothing, and to avoid larger crowds.

Some people advocated for the constant use of oils in

the nose and throat during this time. It was thought that they protected these areas from penetration by the infection. There was, however, no scientific evidence that accompanied this. In general, it was more recommended to practice general oral hygiene as a safer and more established practice.

PUBLIC HEALTH ADMINISTRATION

Following the influenza epidemic, it was clear that the administrative side of Public Health could be modified. First off, centralization of the public health initiatives could distribute health guidelines and policies more effectively. Secondly, standardization of health laws and penalties for all states could ensure uniform compliance. Another modification, and an extremely important one in terms of epidemics, came in the form of reporting infectious diseases. It was recommended by the American Medical Association that any physician who willfully fails to report communicable diseases by struck from their membership. Additionally, gathering information on daily admissions and large population areas could more accurately track and predict outbreaks. These data were recommended to be on file with a person dedicated to these functions. Finally, printed procedures should be recommended for how to deal with isolation in patients suspected of illness.

There were several laws suggested to be implemented in the event of an epidemic. The first of these was provisions for the boards of health to acquire existing vaccines, sera, or other materials when an unusual demand calls for them, and for them to be distributed at the normal price. A second law that was suggested that the boards of health have the power to strike any advertisements containing obviously false information in regard to the epidemic. A third law permitted health authorities to render public eating places to inspection to ensure proper sterilizing techniques. The law allowed for punishment to be implemented for violation of said rules. These laws in essence would give control over the domain of public health to the boards of health in order to cease delay in any sort of essential measures necessary to control an epidemic.

It was suggested that during the times of epidemics that health authorities should trust the public with all accurate information available. This was recommended to start with a general bulletin with all the main facts. During the epidemic this was released by the American Public Health Service, but the distribution method led to it being missed by a large proportion of the population. It was recommended following this failure that newspapers would be used freely in order to facilitate improvement in this category. A question and answer department was postulated to verify facts distributed to the public for the next epidemic. The public was encouraged to come forth with knowledge that could be verified or corrected, so that knowledge of circulating rumors would become apparent to health advisors. This was an issue during the 1918 epidemic, as there were posting of so-called "Sure Cures" that did not have any scientific proof of efficacy. This was also an idea that could allow do-gooders to verify their information and facilitate their desire to spread effective countermeasures to the epidemic. Some anecdotal advice that ended up rising to the surface during the epidemic were placing sulfur in shoes, wearing of amulets, inhaling chloroform, etc., all which rightly should have been prevented from being widely circulated. Distribution of placards with helpful information was an additional benefit to distribute information widely. An additional suggestion that arose was that an authoritative presence in each area should be the spokesperson for boards of health, so that a trusted source could remain in a reliable capacity.

In sum, the prevention of an epidemic where the causative organism is unknown creates a substantial logistical problem moving forward. The known fact that the illness is spread by contact was one of the most important facets of knowledge for prevention of future epidemics, and indeed most of the infrastructure changes were dedicated towards decreasing this method of spread. It was determined that Health Departments should have a preparedness policy that ensures swift and effective actions in order to minimize casualties, and that centralization and standardization of work should be readily able to be enacted so that new findings can be reliable and readily distributed. Physicians were expected to be informed on the various measures that are necessary to treat epidemic patients. Meanwhile, the public should learn the value of remaining well-rested and avoiding public spaces in order to help their fellow man. They should strictly obey public health orders, and all businesses should be ready to accommodate new requirements.

DISCUSSION OF EPIDEMIC INFLUENZA

INSPIRED BY THE WORK OF W. L. HOLMAN, M. D.

Technical difficulties when it comes to respiratory disease are difficult and must be overcome in order to provide accurate results. The important problems include: the study of smears and cultures, tests that determine the causative agent, and studies of real-time infections.

When choosing material to sample in respiratory illness, the difficulty is to pick something that will accurately represent what is causing disease. Any sputum used for growing bacteria was recommended to be obtained from the lowest areas of the respiratory tract, should not have any material from the mouth, and should be washed before use. These were considered the minimum standard for getting a sample. Other methods (blood culture, lung puncture, spinal fluid) have their own protocols for collection.

The methods used to highlight the bacteria growing in culture, since this investigation was focusing only on one bacteria (B. influenzae), focused on using stains that would highlight its presence. The problem with B. Influenzae was that it is exceedingly small and is not always the same shape and size, making it difficult to visualize. Also, the shape of B.

influenzae was very peculiar in that it sometimes comes in pairs and is extremely small. This made identification of the bacteria through the identification of chains pretty common, and also made it complicated somewhat, since a long-curled chain could be misidentified as a bacteria named leptothrix. However, when a good sample was obtained, the odds of an accurate result precipitously increased.

Another problem with culturing bacteria came from the fact that the nutrition required for growth varies widely depending on the type of bacteria, with no universal nutrition that can grow all. The specific method of growing for B. Influenzae used a specialized growth plate that proved consisted enough to rule in or out its presence. They were typically also multiple bacteria that looked similar to B. Influenzae, so this dictated that multiple trials be run to confirm.

Swabs were used in this study from large areas of the lung from 32 autopsies and blood cultures from 22 patients. The express purpose was to isolate the bacteria itself for testing. Most other bacteria found were identified.

Direct smears were made and stained. Cultures were made using specialized growth nutrition and was modified according to the results it produced.

THE HEMOPHILIC BACTERIA

One of the important findings was that B. Influenzae requires hemoglobin, the protein that carries oxygen in red blood cells, to grow. Blood can typically help bacteria grow in the lab as a nutritious substance, but it seemed a necessary component for the bacteria in question. There are few other bacteria who utilize this strategy, but they typically thrive in other types of mammals. This led to the notion that B. Influenzae must have blood for growth. Multiple growth mediums, a term for the nutrient supply to bacteria, had been tested to exploit this fact for growth. Also, the addition of other types of bacteria can bring the influenza bacteria to growth in circumstances where it usually will not grow. This was an important finding; in that it could probably exacerbate the conditions when multiple bacteria are present as well as lead to secondary infection of other kinds of bacteria. The ultimate conclusion to these findings were that the right medium and accompanying bacteria was that B. Influenzae is difficult to grow in laboratory settings. It was mainly expressed to give rise to the notion that in studies where this proper care was not taken, the results should be suspect.

B. Influenzae had some prominence as the causative agent in clinical influenza. Both live and killed cultures placed into animals had a toxic effect. It was also shown that animals with a lowered immune system, performed by deliberate infection, would become infected at a higher rate. After repeated infections from other kinds of bacteria, it was shown in animals that B. influenzae could be lethal on its own. The strains of B. Influenzae recovered from meningitis cases, an infection of the brain, proved to be especially damaging when given to animals. When killed bacteria were used, it showed that it produced toxins that can operate on their own volition. This was important because it was the first time a toxin had been obtained from the bacteria, and the effect of the toxin in animals was remarkably similar to that seen in influenza patients. Identifying a toxin could be more reliable in diagnosing an illness than culture of the bacteria, and thus is an important known fact for diagnosis. Indeed, several findings were indicative of the potency of the bacteria B. influenzae.

Influenza was known to be primarily a respiratory illness, with varying degrees of severity. It was believed to be capable of chronic infections lasting years, to mere days. One of the additional components of this illness that was thought to be not well known was its presence as a complication of other diseases, as well as its prevalence in people who participated as carriers, failing to show any signs of infection. Most patients during the epidemic showed the three to five-day illness of influenza, with occasional further involvement of the respiratory tract and secondary pneumonia. Bed rest was vital to early treatment to prevent severe disease. The lack of evidence suggesting which severity a person would experience influenza made the disease all the more a mystery.

After surveying data, it seemed apparent that the incubation period of the disease was approximately two days. It was thought that a wave of infection passing through any given location would last about six weeks, when it was thought that all members of that community had been exposed by that point. Healthy carriers were thought to be a frequent component of spread. During epidemic years, the percentage of carriers in a given population were around 24-33%, whereas in the subsiding years it fell to around 10%, and during the summer as low as 1.5-3.3%. A study by Tedesko reported results covering the years from 1896-1906 that B. Influenzae is continually present in the population, existing in healthy carriers during times of perceived remission. This finding was confirmed in several other studies that found B. Influenzae in the respiratory tracts of healthy individuals. This finding led to the hypothesis that all persons infected with the bacteria were considered as positive for disease, with the varying degrees of illness considered to be a measure of individual resistance. Also, it seemed that different years carried with them different severities. In 1918, the predominant symptom of influenza was pneumonia. This presentation led to a more severe consequence of the disease, and a relatively high mortality. There was also a note that high mortality years were typically preceded by multiple years of mild outbreaks, which was also consistent with the 1918 outbreak.

The difficulty at which laboratory culture of B. Influenzae was possible led to contradicting results by scientists. From some of the more reliable centers, the prevalence of the bacteria was clearer. A study from Camp MacArthur showed a 76.8% positive sputum rate out of 2,279 suspected cases, but when cultured, the number yielded only 10%. This led to the idea that sputum analysis could be more reliable. Numerous attempts were made to identify the bacteria using samples from the blood as well as other organs, but only samples from the lungs had any sort of reliability. These numbers also seemed to decrease when the sample was at autopsy rather than during life.

The percentage of positive results became even more erratic as more individual institutions attempted to try other methods. One minor advance came from Great Britain, which saw that when the sputum became frothier, the numbers of positive results increased. One group from this area was considering a different bacteria, M. Catarrhalis, to be causative of influenza, and ran a study in which they found this organism in all 50 cases. However, B. Influenzae was also grown in 62% of those cases.

Similar numbers of colonization had been found throughout the world, from Korea to Brazil, France, and Italy, and beyond. It was agreed that B. Influenzae was found frequently in cases of influenza, although the causation was disputed. Some scientists debated that it was a combination of different kinds of bacteria that yielded the illness, namely other types of a bacteria family known as pneumococci. It was also postulated that B. Influenzae only lowered the immune system of the host, and the damage was caused by other existing bacteria. B. infleunzae, however, was the most regularly found organism in the pandemic, with the causes of secondary damage being whatever local flora that population happened to have, since it differs widely among distant areas. The compilation of this research led to the hypothesis that influenza could very well be a mixed infection.

In people with chronic lung conditions, B. Influenzae

was a frequent finding. Often, pulmonary tuberculosis, caused by the bacteria M. Tuberculosis, would have B. Influenzae as a secondary positive result. It was determined at this time that it could not be ruled out as a potential cause of these types of chronic infections and was thought to be an important research point in future outbreaks. However, when it came to active epidemics, this was of little use.

B. Influenzae is commonly recovered in the lining between the lung and the ribcage, known as the pleura. One case even retrieved large amounts of pus from this area, a condition known as empyema, in which the bacteria was cultured.

Sinus infections had long been recognized as a symptom of influenza. The numbers of positive results of B. Influenzae from cultures of these areas varied pretty widely. An interesting theory from Lindenthal was that the bacteria may house in the sinuses of individuals in between outbreaks. This finding was supported by some, but not by others. For those interested in the finding, they also theorized that the presence of the bacteria in the sinuses could lead to more severe disease due to toxin production. However, it was the act of participating in spread that they considered the most important part of this finding, as determining the carrier state of the disease was crucial to its future prevention.

Eye infections due to this bacteria were considered quite common. Numbers as high as 66-90% of influenza patients could have positive results, whereas unaffected patients had a rate of positive results around 5.8%. It was known since 1903 that the bacteria could cause eye infection, and the bacteria was frequently found in secretions of the eye. The middle ear, as well as sinus cavities behind the ear, were known to become infected as well. It was important to note however, that secondary bacteria causing destruction was often a common finding in middle ear infections.

Meningitis caused by B. Influenzae was a universally agreed upon characteristic. However, it was noted that only particular strains of the bacteria could cause it.

INVASION OF THE BLOOD STREAM

A constant feature of influenza was infection of the blood, which led to severe illness of the whole body. It was seen that during the peak of the fever the blood results were most likely to be positive. Samples taken before and after the peak tended to have less success. The 1918 epidemic saw infrequent positive blood tests, which argued against the evidence of blood invasion. Scientists familiar with the process were quick to note that the amount of blood used for testing was often less than half what was typically used when the positive result correlation was established. They also noted the difficulty in growth for inexperienced labs as a factor. Nevertheless, even with accurate testing, it was known that the presence of the bacteria in the blood was only transient even during the illness. Future testing on this subject was thought to revolve around identifying different strains that caused different types of illness.

Endocarditis, which is an infection of the lining of the heart, is frequently seen in association with B. influenzae. In fact, it was the second most common bacteria found in these cases in blood testing, after an organism named strepto-cocci. The appendix is also a frequent organ that is found to have B. Influenzae colonization. The bacteria can also infect the gallbladder, testes, and urinary tract. This was evidence that, although primarily a respiratory pathogen, B. Influenzae knew no bounds when infecting the body.

Ingestion of B. influenzae by immune cells was very frequently noted when they were looked at under the microscope. This is most prevalent when patients were in recovery.

Agglutination, or, the tendency of cells to clump together, was an area of interest in regard to this bacteria. The difficulty with this is that most secondary infections will cause this reaction in the blood, leading to tedious work determining the cause. The agglutination rate was increased in people after the peak of the disease and to those vacci-nated against the bacteria. Most importantly, it was a differing quality between strains of the bacteria, so that it could potentially be used for identification.

The complement pathway, which is a component of the immune system comprised of binding proteins, showed a positive binding correlation when serum was taken from patients at the end of their illness, usually about 3-5 days following but as long as 45 days after. Acutely ill patients saw a substantially lower amount of complement until they started to recover. This seemed to indicate immune response to the infection.

There was an interesting theory that the outbreaks of the illness were due to prior sensitization of populations to the mild forms, and then a severe reaction to a recurrence, much like an allergy. This very quickly was debunked, however.

WAVE OF INFLUENZA

The Influenza Pandemic led to a large expansion of human testing in medicine. There were over 200 men who volunteered to be injected with pure cultures of bacteria. Despite this act of altruism, the results yielded little in terms of discerning the transmission of the disease. The fact of the matter was, following the pandemic in 1918, there was truly little known about how influenza spread so rapidly. B. Influenzae proved a promising target, but there was not enough evidence to conclude what caused this rash of illness on the world.

Influenza spread through the Military Hospital in Pittsburgh in 1918 provided a time of massive amounts of data collection, lasting about five weeks, that was extremely valuable for real-time evaluation of the components of an epidemic. This section will take each part of the body and discuss the effects that influenza has on that part of the body. There is a large amount of material to discuss even as it is restricted by these criteria, so that it will inform how influenza affects the body. It will dive into the progression of the disease how it is seen in clinics and hospitals, from early to late events, as it was known during this time. There are plenty of differences depending on surrounding area, region, and population, which will also be appreciated to shine more light on any possible associations. These observations will be made within the context of the height of an epidemic, from individuals who died from the disease, in which there was definitely evidence of a lung infection process. This involves 639 patients admitted to the hospital during this time, of which 35 died. All the individuals were from military camps, were enrolled in the army, and were ages 18-30 in good physical condition.

There were no consistent external characteristics that could clearly be pointed to as a mark of influenza. Lack of oxygen (cyanosis), which turns the skin blue, was seen in the face, head, neck, and shoulders commonly, but not enough to be universal. Of these cases, it was always the upper part of the body that had this trait, with the face always being the most affected, particularly the lips and ears. This was a common sign in ordinary pneumonia as well. Some places where the lack of oxygen was also evident was the fingertips under the nails, more so in the upper extremities than the lower. There was no evidence of swelling that came with this. One patient had a rash on the chest, which looked like pinpoint purplish dots. There were occasional skin lesions that seemed to be the start of boils or pustules, which were common post-influenza symptoms. It was thought that this could indicate presence of influenza in the surrounding tissues.

There were two cases where there were burst blood vessels in the eyes. They were both limited to one eye. One case also had yellowing of the eye and skin: a symptom commonly seen in liver damage. This patient had corresponding liver damage.

There were no kidney issues with any of the patients. Interestingly, in the 1890 epidemic in Canada, there was substantial kidney damage. These individuals also had swelling, of which was not present in the Pittsburgh subjects. Swelling is a known sign of kidney damage, which is worth note.

Almost all of these patients were in the best of health due to their military training, which was a striking realization. In 14 of the 32 patients autopsied, damage to the abdominal muscles was sustained. Tearing of this muscle was frequent in these patients, mostly at the middle of the muscle. A complete tear was usually in the lower portion of the abdominals. There was often accompanying bleeding that would be expected with the amount of blood flow that usually went to these areas. Similar findings were expressed in the chest muscles, but to a much less degree, with only two patients showing evidence.

Since one feature of influenza is muscular weakness, it was interesting to correlate these findings. Originally it was thought that weakness in an individual was caused by lack of energy, but there is a plausible hypothesis with these findings that there is actual damage to the muscle. Microscopic examination of muscle showed that it was not an inflammatory process by the body that caused this, and that it was purely carried out by a toxic process, of which influenza was known to produce. The damage was limited to specific portions of skeletal muscle, with preference for some over others. Moreover, the muscle often retained its normal shape, but staining showed clear weakness, indicating that it was probable that the damage was not caused by mechanical movement. It followed many of the same characteristics of muscle damage in typhoid fever, which shows a waxy change. This change is accompanied by degenerated fibers that eventually turn to waste that builds up in the muscle. Scar tissue starts to build in proportion to the damage done, especially in areas of heavy bleeding. These could partially account for the abdominal pain seen in influenza, which is often not attributed to any specific organ. It could very well be likely that damage to the abdominal wall muscles is what causes this.

The majority of individuals had few visible lesions in the nose, mouth, or throat. Some had complained of throat dryness prior to death, but there were no evident causes of this. Congestion of the nose was much milder than similar respiratory diseases, but bleeding was still common during the acute illness. Causes of nose bleed were not found, and it was thought to be unusual the lack of running noses in the population. Also, while some patients complained of hoarseness, which was then found to be caused by swelling of the larynx (voice box), this finding was not consistent. It was below the vocal cords that the real evidence of a respiratory illness began.

All 32 cases showed inflammation of the trachea (commonly known as the windpipe). There was substantive evidence of acute inflammation, with a thin layer of film lining the surface. The trachea could also be found to be filled with a frothy fluid, which had more reserve deeper in the lung. Damage to the mucus lining of the trachea was evident, which was important because of its ability to give access to the organism to the tissue below it (mucus normally provides a protective barrier to surfaces). The trachea was found to be intensely inflamed, however, there was only one case where dead tissue was found. This was the most striking finding and was not paralleled by infectious process of any other cause. It often was continuous all the way down to the airway portions of the lung. It was thought that this was how the illness spread, from trachea downward.

Additional features of the trachea inflammation included backed up blood vessels and hemorrhaging, stretching of spaces in between tissues, and local swelling limited to this region. This led to damage of the lining of the trachea, as all the contents leaked out into the area. In the patients autopsied, this process seemed further along, with larger areas of damage to the lining. This led to swelling of the inner portions of the trachea. Damaging processes occurred to nearby areas as blood vessels and cells leaked their contents. However, interestingly, there was still very few areas of dead tissue. Blood clots were common in the small blood vessels of the area, indicating a distinct characteristic of this illness. This was suspected to also be the case in the lower areas of the lung, which would make breathing more difficult.

Another change demonstrated in this area was in reference to the lymphatic system, which controls the drainage of all waste made by cells and is a route for immune cells to follow. These channels typically were found to be enlarged with fluid, and later with immune cells called lymphocytes. This is typically a response to invasion.

The amount and characteristics of the thin film lining the trachea was correlated to the extent of the illness. Underneath this layer and the lining of the trachea, differences in injury could also be observed to determine disease severity. The mucus glands seemed to have no role in the inflammatory process which may be due to over secretion and subsequent protection from invasion. This could be partly how the lung protects itself.

The lesions seen in the bronchi, which are the continuations of the trachea into each individual lung, were very much a continuation of the findings seen in the trachea. The amount of inflammation seen in the trachea is very comparable to that in the upper airway. As the track progresses downward, these findings generally become milder, and it was thought that the change in material facilitated this (lower airway is more composed of muscle, versus cartilage, with more lymphatic drainage).

The loss of the lining of the bronchi is consistent with that of the trachea where the infection seems to be present. The progression of loss of lining to immune system infiltration is also consistent. In the smallest parts of the lung, termed the bronchioles, the inflammation only becomes present when the disease has clearly overtaken that area of the lung. The muscles of these areas show evidence of degeneration, consistent with the muscular degeneration found in other areas of the body. This can lead to destruction of the air-passing sacs known as alveoli, which usually fill up with air on inhalation and compress on exhalation. If they are destroyed, they remain open and unable to participate in gas exchange, leading to less active lung that can get oxygen into the bloodstream. There was often copious amounts of mucus inside the bronchi in most cases, but destruction of gas-exchanging areas of the lungs happened in only 4. However, there had been existing reports that, even without destruction of the lung tissue, a certain percentage of people recovering from influenza never regained full function of their affected lungs.

The deeper parts of the lung were quite easy to identify when they became infected, as they were intensely inflamed and often had pus on their surface. The enlarged blood vessels were also quite easy to visualize. It was unclear, however, how deep the infection had to occur for permanent damage to be sustained. It was evident that the deeper the infection went, ; the more nearby areas of the lung were affected. However, a point of no return had not been documented. It was thought that this inflammatory reaction was responsible for the most damage that the disease caused.

Smaller airways within the lung were often more easily affected than the larger ones. Involvement of these airways often caused a condition similar to pneumonia. In fact, some of these airways could be infected even without their higher up counterparts showing any signs of a similarly intense reaction. It is important to note, however, that it was not possible to tell if involvement of the deeper areas of the lung came before or after higher airways were involved, in the case of pneumonia-like conditions. In some cases, groups of bacteria growing together, termed an abscess, would be found at the deep parts of the lung.

The recovery process of these parts of the lung were difficult to observe since the patients never recovered from illness. There was some evidence that the body attempted to repair damaged areas with connective tissue. The amount of connective tissue made in some instances could have restricted air flow to that area of lung, which would cause shortness of breath to the individual. It was assumed that those individuals who recovered without loss of lung function preserved enough of their normal lung tissue to regenerate it in the normal way that the lung replaces cells. In the few cases where patients were autopsied outside of this study after they had overcome influenza, the lungs appeared normal 5-6 weeks following resolution.

Although many parts of the body can be affected by influenza, there was no doubt that no person suffered a fatal illness without a lesion in the lung. Therefore it is important to understand the effect this disease has on the lung to determine what happens after the fact. There are complications that can arise (abscesses, pneumonia, tissue death), but the main assault on the lung is carried out by the disease itself. The complicating aspect, however, is that the effect influenza has on the lung is not always consistent. Therefore, descriptions of epidemics vary widely in what is considered a primary infection of the illness. Additionally, this illness cannot be replicated in animal models, and those who come to autopsy have a high rate of mixed infection causing mortality, which almost always is a complication after the disease has occurred. This section will try to use the data gathered from Pittsburgh to come up with a uniform and detailed description of how the lungs are affected. A study by Dr. Holman in 1893 on 40 patients will also be used to round out some of the data.

The acute stages of influenza is distinctive enough so that it cannot be misunderstood as pneumonia. This is not based off of a single finding, but a host of findings, which include the type of injury to the lung, its character, the extent of the lung involved, and the multiple stages of recovery that the lung expresses. Injury to the lung usually occurs in four stages: congestion, red hepatization, gray hepatization, and resolution. Normal pneumonia is rarely found in the first two stages as they happen too quickly. In influenza, however, most of the lungs are found in this state. Additionally, pneumonia tends to affect only one lobe of the lung at a time (the right lung possesses 3 lobes, the left 2) at a fairly uniform and expectable rate. These lobes, when affected, will be at the same stage of injury. Influenza, however, tends to have patchy areas throughout the lung, often multiple lobes, affected. Lastly, pneumonia tends to be a dry process, whereas influenza has a high amount of mucus and swelling within the lung. This is what gives way to the term influenza-pneumonia, which is a very distinct and unique process.

The progression of influenza-pneumonia was able to be elicited from the data. The earliest sign was congestion, followed by swelling, small bleeding, and immune system involvement. At this point, the tissue would start to heal or become overwhelmed and die. Most cases where the patient died did so during the first three stages, evident by the lack of any lung healing. Surprisingly, a large proportion of these died during the first stage, which would be unusual in other lung injuries. It was difficult to determine how long this process would take, as in influenza, the stage where the lung was congested was very variable. Using the start of the illness, however, it was suggested that the progression took somewhere around five days. Of note, the amount of lung volume involved was often not enough to compromise the amount of air a person could get to induce death, meaning that there must have been an acute process contributing to this not evident at autopsy.

The height of illness seemed to come when all three of the first stages: congestion, swelling, and hemorrhage, were present. Sometimes, there could be several larger bleeds in the area. These areas of lung would often retain air, although they were likely unusable. It was thought that the amount of fluid in the lungs prevented this air from being transmitted to the bloodstream. The lower lobes were more commonly involved in collection of immune cells and hemorrhage blood. They would take on a "waterlogged" appearance at autopsy that could be molded to different shape.

Some of the bleeding occurred in distinct punctate areas, resembling that of plague pneumonia. They varied in size from walnut to golf ball and could be starkly different in appearance from other areas of the lung. The greater the amount of blood, the less air was typically found in those areas. Of interesting note, the two largest hemorrhages seen were two patients that deteriorated very rapidly and died within 48 hours of lung symptoms.

An important component of influenza in the lungs, it was found that there were multiple areas of lung in affected patients that were at different levels of involvement. This meant that the disease had the capability to continue to injure the lung after the initial insult. Indeed, in all autopsied cases, there were still areas of lung early on in injury, suggesting that the process was actively causing new harm at death.

The swelling seen in the lungs during this illness was well thought to be caused by the body's inflammatory response to an enemy. There are several different kinds of fluids that can fill the lungs. This fluid was clear to be involved via an inflammatory process. Although blood was present in all of the swelling samples, it was thought that the blood components were not part of the swelling response but merely an artifact that was impossible to keep separate during lab harvest. This was important because it differentiated this type of swelling from that seen in heart and kidney disease, which has other characteristics. This fluid could also be mixed with blood, which the patient, while alive, to cough up quite a bit of, enough to lose up to a pint of blood at a time.

The earliest insult to the lung found, which was distinct for influenza pneumonia, involved a wet lung with blood-stained fluid, with no evidence that the lung had advanced past the first two stages of injury. The stage that was absent, red hepatization, only occurs when certain substances are mixed inside of it and is characteristic of lobar pneumonia.

When the lungs were examined microscopically, the damage was consistent with the rapid effect influenza was thought to have on them. Blood vessels were widened as far as they were capable, and there was marked swelling between cells in the air-filling sacs (termed alveoli). Tissue within the lung was distended and bogged down. This happened much more quickly than in standard pneumonia. The absence of a protein called fibrin, which aids in forming blood clots, was also noted, which is an expressly unique characteristic to influenza pneumonia.

Swelling was often accompanied by various amounts of bleeding in the alveoli. The open blood vessel could often be found, and usually did not affect the ability of the lung to continue to receive blood. It suggested an acute process leading to a break in the blood vessel wall, but no mechanism of action could be found. When blood was around for a while, different types of cells were found in small amounts, as well as cells known as mononuclear cells, which exist to clean up dead cells by ingesting them. Another cell known as a macrophage, which is a larger version of the mononuclear cell, would often follow.

The inflammatory reaction cause by the illness would often impact the alveoli. There was often a cartilage-like substance called hyaline found in the swelling that was of unknown use but came attached to the walls of the sacs and is known to become available following damage to the lining. These clumps of hyaline could often block vessels and lead to death of the area. These blockages led some people to believe it serves the same purpose as fibrin, but the majority of data led to the opposite conclusion. It was agreed upon, however, that the presence of this substance indicated a particularly severe injury to the lower lungs.

Broadly incorporating all of these findings, it was

evident that the influenza pneumonia in early stage was characterized by rapid inflammation and hemorrhage. It is during this phase where the bacteria are shown within the lung, but not at a uniform level. They very much exist in different areas than those of injured lung. This would be left for further inquiry.

The second stage of lung damage, following the inflammation and local swelling, comes at variable times. This stage of lung injury in influenza is more similar to ordinary pneumonia and is accompanied by some fibrin and cells. The lung loses some weight from fluid leaving the area, and changes to a paler color. This is termed gray consolidation. It is difficult to recognize the start of this process because the bleeding from the acute stage sticks around for some time even after it is no longer active. Indeed, the lung can be in a full secondary stage without being apparent to the naked eye. Once the new material hits a threshold, the color change becomes evident. The earliest this was seen was during the 4th day of infection, with the majority happening more towards the 6th day and some as late as the 8th. This stage represents some level of progression of response by the body to influenza.

Although the gray consolidation looks similar to normal pneumonia, the distribution within the lung clearly separates it from the same process. It is consistent with the original injury of influenza, in that it appears patchy and throughout the lung, instead of limited to one or two lobes. This type of distribution is only seen in one other type of pneumonia, that which follows measles infection. In this type of pneumonia, there is patchy involvement, but the patches are round and small with smooth edges, not like that of influenza, which is very irregular, almost leaf-like. It also is made up of wet sticky fluid, which is rarely seen in pneumonia, a typically dry process. In fact, this consistency actually resembles active pneumonia more closely before the lung is recovering.

The differing stages of recovery was also characteristic of influenza over other forms of pneumonia. The stages of recovery of each affected area of the lung can be different, even within the same lobe or right next to each other. The gray stage is seen first more frequently in the lower lobes of the lung, very often starting with the upper portion of the right lower lobe. This is often the area of the lung that is affected first in normal pneumonia, which is an interesting fact of note.

This type of progression seemed to vary depending on location. Some other areas described some other processes such as involvement of the lining of the lung and stated that the affected areas in the lung were multiple and small, much more the size of a small pea. This process seemed to progress differently than the type of influenza injury seen in Pittsburgh but was more closely resembling post-measles pneumonia. It was postulated that the different types of influenza pneumonia outside the standard process that was described above could be due to associated infection with other kinds of bacteria, namely those of the streptococcus family.

The lack of distribution to one or two lobes of the lung is a logical reason why the physical exam findings were difficult to elucidate in influenza. Typically, in pneumonia, when one entire lobe is in recovery and not functioning, that changes the breath sounds that can be heard with a stethoscope. When this recovery is not uniform, there are enough breath sounds to complicate the findings, to the point where it could be missed on physical exam that a portion of lung is affected.

Once this gray stage sets in, the lung becomes soft and easily bleeds, a characteristic known as friability. Tissue can easily be broken if handled, much like that of dry clay. This was thought to be because most of the lung tissue was damaged and would not have its normal fortitude against mechanical stress. Additionally, abscesses (areas of bacteria enclosed by connective tissue) could have been present that gives the false impression of solid tissue but is rather dead space. These combinations lead to easily injured lung tissue.

One of the questions posed during this gray stage is whether the lung is susceptible to a second infection by another bacteria. Based on evaluation of the bacteria present, it was unable to be determined whether the lung was in an early phase of recovery or in the beginning of a secondary pneumonia. Indeed, both of these processes could look identical. Since influenza causes damage so rapidly, it could be this vulnerable state of the lung that other types of bacteria take advantage of. This could be a reason why the lung injury is irregular and at different stages, as it could be the degree to which other types of bacteria extend the injury. In tissue where secondary injury has possibly occurred, these are the areas that in some instances never recover.

During this secondary stage of lung infection, there is an intense immune response, noted by the amount of pus that occupies the lung. This can at some places stop the blood supply due to the volume of immune cells in the blood vessels, which can lead to small areas of tissue death around them. In the larger airways (bronchi), there were observations of areas where the wall had become weak, and even destroyed.

The lymphatic drainage system of the lungs were found to be active during this stage, allowing for draining of material that no longer served function in the lung. There were several immune cells scattered about this system, which were known to usually only become active when there is disturbance to the structure of the lung. These cells were also found in the sputum.

Because of these differences, it was wondered whether pneumonia was the proper term, or what the proper term should be, for lung injury caused by influenza. It was apparent from the areas of the lung that were seen to be injured that the geographic location was too variable to be used to name this type of illness. Additionally, it would not be able to capture the inflammatory process which was the most damaging part. It was believed that the early phases of the infection, the inflammatory phase, was that which was most consistent and worthy of attention. The secondary injury, in contrast, had too many variables, and was often attributed to too many types of secondary bacteria, to be used in nomenclature. These secondary bacteria were differing depending on geographical location, so while it would be helpful for each practitioner to know their regional secondary bacteria for treatment, they would not be helpful in diagnosis. Additionally, the appearance of pus occurred too late to be considered as a useful area of diagnosis. There was even enough dispute to the causative organism that it could not be used for definitive diagnosis. It was believed that the kinds of pneumonia, if they could be put into a few categories, could be useful to direct treatment. However, the causes could not be linked to any population characteristics that would be reliable. The presence of streptococcus bacteria was the most consistent in its secondary infection, but this can only be determined after the primary insult. Thus, the categorization of influenza pneumonia was still left in question after this study.

The clearance of inflammation and return to normal function was carried out very slowly by the body. This stage rarely found any sort of complications and was found to begin usually around the 10th-12th day of illness. Each area of recovery in the lung was proportional to the amount of injury that was caused. In areas where swelling was the only process, simply the natural drainage of the body was enough to return the lung to normal. It was thought that in these areas, there was no damage that allowed secondary bacteria to get a hold of tissues underneath the lining. These areas required no further repair.

Interestingly, as acute as the induction of the influenza illness happens, it was equally quick to disappear. The latter stages of recovery appear to be resolved more quickly than the evidence of the recovery is seen by the lung. The lack of repairing material evident in the swelling fluid of the lung in influenza led people to believe that the natural draining of the swelling is enough to return undamaged portions of the lung to their normal state. However, when portions of the lung were damaged, recovery was not as simple. It would be difficult to determine areas of complete recovery on autopsy if they were not unique to normal lung tissue. However, in most known cases, damage to the tissue of the lung does not return to a form that is indistinguishable. The presence of minuscule blood clots, repair tissue, or bacterial abscesses all indicated injury during illness. This type of resolution can only be accomplished by scar tissue connecting the damaged areas, with the amount being proportional to the size of the damage. This repair seemed to be quicker than what was expected, in some cases scar tissue being accomplished in as little as 23 days after illness. This arrival often was corresponding with the loss of pus in the area. However, these areas seemed unable to return to their normal function. If this area was substantial, the patient often had shortness of breath that was accordingly proportional.

A type of repair that is less permanent, termed granulation, was often seen earlier during the gray phase of lung injury. This type of repair is more transient, and if successful, could restore normal function to the area. This was a crucial part of lung recovery; in that it could preserve the function of the lung.

If the blood supply to an area of the lung was occluded to a large degree, these areas would experience tissue death. This type of death would result in a cream white color, thought to be a mixture of pus and dead tissue, that eventually would disintegrate.

One of the effects that is substantial in influenza was the fact that it damages not only the functional areas of the lung, but the connecting tissue between them. This was evidence that it can be capable of a total lung injury. Pus was found in all areas of the lung, including the muscles, and connecting tissue. This appeared to be toxic damage when referring to the areas between the functional parts of the lung, due not to an invasion of the organism itself but by a toxin it produces.

The summary of all of these effects on the lung are that, unfortunately the effects of influenza pneumonia is both complex and inconsistent. Resolution may be quick and more efficient than could be observed if there was no damage to the lining or may be delayed if the immune system became involved. It commonly affects the areas of the lung in an unpredictable pattern, and is gone often as quickly as it came, leaving a potential site for secondary infection. The majority of cases seem to experience complete healing or a minor amount of scarring, but if persistent, can end up with a complicated illness. Those who start to recover before invasion of the immune system begins tended to have the best outcome.

The pleura, which is a lining over the outer lung, was an important consideration for any respiratory illness. In respect to influenza, as with most things, it was variable and unpredictable. The scientific community agreed that there was an interval in between when the lung was involved and when the pleura became inflamed. There were 27 cases in the Pittsburgh study where the pleura became inflamed, though it was not determined whether these could have been evident in clinic, as these were included even if they were the slightest reaction. The reactions varied from the smallest amount of swelling to acute and involved scarring.

The most common involvement of this lining was an increase in the fluid caught by the lining. This quantity varied, and was usually clear, although it was not uncommon to be contaminated with some blood. This seemed to occur early on in the inflammation stage of the illness and were mostly well contained. Bleeding from the pleura itself only became apparent during severe cases. When hemorrhage did occur, it was typically on the posterior areas of the lower lobes. When bacteria was able to invade this space, the fluid would become much cloudier, and have accompanying immune cells. This bacteria was almost always resembling the type of bacteria that was normally present in lung.

When the pleura became involved late in the disease course, it was very typically filled with pus and immune contents, termed empyema. Interestingly, later cases of this did not show any B. Influenzae bacteria, which was consistent with the absence of the bacteria in late stages of the disease. The epidemic of 1918 saw a rise in these type of cases found in surgery following the wave of illness. However, hardly any of the autopsy cases found substantial involvement. It was also assumed as well, with the rapid infectious capability of the illness, that the involvement of the pleura could be resolved by the time it was available for evaluation.

During the height of the epidemic, there was hardly any involvement of the heart. The only cases where the lining of the heart was colonized by bacteria were seemingly correlated with secondary infection rather than influenza itself. Like the lining of the lung, the fluid that surrounded the hard in the few cases where it did was clear and very minimal. There was some very minor bleeding in the heart, which could have been indicative of toxin spread from the lung in small amounts. There was only case where there was enough damage of the heart to weaken its muscle, and it was unable to be determined if the patient had a preexisting heart condition.

Any of the minor damage that occurred in the heart seemed to resolve without any lasting scarring. There were no relationships between heart lesions and influenza infection. Some mild swelling was present, which was common in many infections. The interesting note of this was the lack of damage to muscle in the heart. As noted in previous sections, the influenza illness tended to have a degenerating effect on skeletal muscles. The heart is composed of a different type of muscle and was seemingly unaffected. It was thought that some difference in the two tissues led to the heart being spared.

In a few cases, there were accumulations of growth of bacteria, termed vegetations, in small quantities on the mitral valve. It did not appear that it affected the function in any way.

In order to expand on these findings, enough information from over 400 autopsies was compiled. Only one of these studies found any effect on the heart, and it was later determined that the patients in this study had a dormant tuberculosis infection. This could have been a combinatory effect, although it was generally more accepted that there was no overt heart damage caused by influenza.

Since the Pittsburgh study focused on young adults, the shape of the arteries was remarkably healthy. However, in most, there was evidence of damage to the aorta, the largest blood vessel leaving the heart, which was believed to be related to the cause of death. This was present in 28 of the 32 cases. This damage was striking, and similar to that caused by heart disease, which was extremely unusual given the age of the subjects. They existed only on the back wall of the aorta in the form of fatty layers and could extend as far as the blood vessels in the neck. These lesions would not have been enough to block blood flow from the heart, but they served as an indicator that there was some sort of acute process occurring that led to their formation. These had only been previously seen as a consequence of high cholesterol. One interesting difference in these lesions of influenza were that they existed only on the surface of the inner blood vessel, where in heart disease they usually extend deeper. In animal subjects these had been known to appear and then disappear, but since these patients were deceased, that could not be observed.

It appeared that these fatty streaks developed as some sort of consequence of alteration of cholesterol metabolism in the body. This could have occurred in the blood, adrenal glands, or liver. In these three tissues, alterations by bacterial toxins can cause fatty streaks. The cells of the blood vessels are particularly good at taking up the excess cholesterol in these cases. However, for them to remain on the surface was unusual. Damage to the blood vessels deeper than the surface was not observed.

There were occasional reports that blood clots formed following influenza illness. They were diverse in area and could have possibly been related to materials put into the bloodstream by muscle degeneration. In cases of the lung, these blood clots were formed by infection immediately surrounding them and did not show the normal materials used for standard blood clots. The clots that formed were more typically in the veins than arteries. In any case, it was unknown what to make of this finding.

The lymphatic system, which was previously mentioned to be the drainage system of cellular waste in the body, was a highly active component in influenza. The lymph system in the chest was remarkably larger than would be expected in standard pneumonia. These changes seemed to be due to inflammatory substances inside of the channels. These changes were not observed elsewhere in the body, meaning the lymphatic involvement was likely kept to the chest. These changes were observed more quickly than standard pneumonia as well. Blood was found often in the lymphatic system when bleeding in the lungs was involved, likely as an incidental mixture. All the lymphatic tissue around the lungs was enlarged, indicating that they were receiving a large amount of material during the infection.

In response to pathogenic organisms, the lymph system often grows in size at weigh stations known as lymph nodes. This was also evident in influenza, although when these areas were cut open and observed, there were so many different kinds of bacteria that it was impossible to determine the cause. It was believed that B. Influenzae could be considered as a cause. These parts of the lymph system were very dilated, often with the same type of fluid seen in the lung swelling. Occasionally, immune cells could also be found in the fluid, particularly when there was pus inside the lungs. When this occurred, the areas where pus was found in the lung corresponded to the areas where it was found in the drainage system. When the lymph nodes were found to possess this material, the infection was very well controlled in the surrounding tissues. Only one case described a scarring of the lymphatic channels, which was seen only previously as a response to streptococcus bacterial infection. This was not thought to be a consequence of influenza.

In the later stages of illness, the lymphatics became filled with yellowish contents that were thicker than the inflammatory fluid. The distribution of this type of fluid was irregular, and often in relation to more affected areas.

It seemed obvious that the important role of drainage by the lymphatic system was evident in influenza pneumonia. This served as an obvious route to which the fluid found in the lungs was allowed to be removed and returned to circulation, as well as where immune cells could travel to fight the infection. This system seemed to adequately handle the stress put on it by the rapid induction of inflammation by influenza.

Evidence that other organs were affected by influenza outside of the lungs was quite scarce and less lethal in nature. It was thought that any damages were the result of toxin spread throughout the body. These could result in small hemorrhages, seen in the stomach, intestines, and bladder, or directly impairing the cells, as in liver and kidney tissue. The absence of inflammation in these areas led to the conclusion that this was likely not being caused by living bacteria, which can be found in the case of some infections, known as bacteremia. Since bacteria in the blood had been shown in influenza, this could not be completely ruled out, but the lack of consistent inflammation of other organs made this an unlikely cause.

In the stomach and intestines, the damage came in two forms: hemorrhage and erosions, or destruction of lining. The stomach showed 15 cases of small bleeds, the intestines 4. These were enough to be found in stool in 12 cases. However, they were not a forceful enough bleed to be concerning and were always small vessels. The erosions that occurred were typically small and round and limited to the top layer of surface. These were likely caused by loss of blood flow to the area. Multiple erosions were found in 10 cases, with the largest being 1.25cm. It was thought that these would likely have healed on their own accord.

In the liver, some moderate swelling was observed in 13 of the 32 cases. One of these cases was enough to cause some mild dysfunction. This led to the idea that the yellowing of the skin and eyes seen in the few cases it was came as a product of bursting blood cells instead of liver dysfunction. The gallbladder and bile ducts were unaffected. In some cases, there were small areas of tissue death in the liver.

The spleen showed only 2 cases where it was enlarged. However, inflammation was diagnosed in 14 cases. These cases appeared to have a spleen that was congested and swollen, and in one case led to bleeding.

The analysis of the kidney was similar to what was expected based on the symptoms, since there was no component of urinary changes in influenza. The amount of urine was slightly decreased, and the color slightly darker. There was only one case where there was urinary obstruction enough to cause any damage. Swelling of the kidneys was common and often very minimal. They did at times seem congested but did not have the presence of any bacteria. Thus, it was thought that these changes were due to a toxin. There were also no changes to the blood vessels in this area. At the conclusion of this, it was thought that kidney damage was not a substantial component of influenza.

Two cases found lesions in the bladder of the subjects. These patients were noted to have blood-stained urine for days prior to their death. The hemorrhages found in the bladder on their death were concordant to those found in the lungs, stomach, and intestine. It was only the bladder, however, that these became large pools of blood. There was no bacteria found in these lesions, which were also assumed to be caused by the toxin.

14 cases saw changes in the adrenal gland, most commonly swelling. The tissue changed from golden in its normal state to brown or clay-colored, with the loss of distinction between its three layers. These were similarly seen in typhoid fever patients. It was thought that this kind of change was a more general response to infection than influenza specific. It was thought that, since the adrenals do store cholesterol to some extent, that this could be the origin of the fatty streaks found in the aorta. However, this hypothesis was not elaborated on, only theorized.

OBSERVATIONS OF EIGHTEEN CASES OF INFLUENZA

This final publication, by J.W. McMeans, offered additional autopsy studies following the 1918 epidemic of influenza. This study also found wet lungs in influenza with the primary component of swelling. The fluid would vary in color and consistency depending on where the lung was at in terms of infection and recovery. Occasionally blood would leak during examination. The only blood vessels affected, consistent with other studies, were small ones. The distribution was concordantly strikingly irregular.

The gray period of lung injury was found to be also present in this study, and the fluid was also changed to a stickier, more mucus in consistency. Abscesses were found in two cases, in which there was extensive tissue death. There were interesting findings of yellow patches on the pleura (lining of the lung) in advanced cases, some so extensive that it looked as if it impeded function. This was only likened to a process where the lymphatic system becomes overwhelmed.

In one case, a large blood clot was found in the lower left

lobe. This area had a surrounding area of tissue death and hemorrhage. There were several surrounding small blood vessels with the yellow clots that have been described previously. It was likely that this was some sort of mixture of immune tissue, mucus, and hyaline.

The presence of different stages of illness within the same lung was also found in these studies. Most frequently, the congestion and inflammatory stage was found to be universal when found, and that when the secondary stages of lung injury occurred, they progressed at their own pace. Almost all cases were found to follow the medium-sized airways (bronchi).

One finding that differed in this study somewhat found that there was an accumulation of fluid in the areas beneath the lungs (known as the pleural cavities). The type of fluid differed depending on the patient, likely due to what stage of lung injury they were in. In almost all cases, both lungs were involved.

The most common systemic (present in the whole body) finding was that of the small bleeds, especially on surfaces of the intestinal tract. The only other consistent finding was swelling of the liver and, to a lesser extent, the spleen. It was concluded from this paper that the hemorrhages were a definite consequence of this illness, the lungs, stomach, and intestinal tract being particularly susceptible. The findings of muscle degeneration were also found here.

This study concluded by stating that influenza caused both a systemic illness and especially injury to the lungs and respiratory tract. It was agreed that the more body wide effects were likely caused by some sort of toxin, while the injury to the respiratory tract likely inflammation, and secondarily, infection by a bacteria following injury. It was agreed in this paper that most cases of fatality would do so during the first 48 hours of infection. The finding of effect on skeletal muscle, particularly the abdominals, was an equally surprising and agreeable report with this study and others. The sparing of the heart and kidney was also perplexing but confirmed by this study.

AUTHOR'S NOTE

After participation in the research for this project, the striking thing of the parallels between the 1918 influenza epidemic and the current coronavirus outbreak of 2020 was how little has changed in regard to response. The theories proposed during this time to improve nationwide response to such an epidemic were useful gleans of information. It seems as though several important factors contributed to how the public and governmental systems respond to such a threat, as will be elaborated below.

First, the common variable that led to similar responses was the lack of an identifiable enemy. In the case of influenza, the culprit was unknown, while in the case of corona, it is poorly understood, amounting to the same presenting information. This leads to a two-sided approach in categorization and documentation. On the public health side, it cannot be overstated how quick identification of the method that the pathogen spreads is of utmost importance.

There are no cases of global health threats by an organism that cannot be stopped by ceasing the passage from one individual to another. This is the front line of defense. However, when the presentation of the disease is unclear, and testing on uncertain grounds, knowing who has the illness becomes cloudy and makes documentation of the spread impossible. This is where the clinical aspect of research is vital. Proper diagnosis of illness must be swift and accurate. If false positives are recorded as cases, the chain of infectivity will lead to substantial amounts of money leading to a path with no resolution. If prevention of spread is the number one goal of public health, accurate diagnosis is the clinical side of that coin. In regard to both of these outbreaks, although signs of infection were unique, an accurate testing method was incomplete, leaving both physicians and health administrators playing shorthanded. Since epidemics usually come from novel sources, this has to be a scenario that is prepared for, given that it is impossible to always know the next outbreak.

Secondly, the distribution of accurate information and discrediting of that which is false is a real-time occupation that carries significant weight for public participation in what must be accomplished. For similar reasons, this seems unchanged between the two epidemics. In the case of 1918, the speed at which information could be distributed was slow and incomplete, leading individuals to resort to more anecdotal and homeopathic information as they sit worried about their fate. In the case of 2020, conversely, information spreads much too quickly, and comes from areas such as social media that are far too easy to be portrayed as holding scientific standing, where they are often no more than riffs of anecdotal evidence. Although it is natural for communities to look for a unified and trusted source that naturally rises to the top, given the technological means in 2020, this was far too poorly executed. Especially since this was suggested to have a universal spokesperson delivering factual information over 100 years ago, the degree to which this has been accomplished is simply unacceptable and leads to civil unrest amongst communities. This was an area where we as a community simply have to be better.

Finally, one of the important jobs in an epidemic, although not useful for the current cases, is close categorization and study of the consequences as they become apparent. Indeed, the most useful aspect of history is to identify its trend in the future. This should have a dedicated institution to studying these effects, as often, unfortunately, there is no shortage of angles from which an epidemic should be analyzed. A scientific paper in 2020 can save thousands of lives in 2050 if it provides even the slightest glean of information to which preventative medicine can move forward.

In closing, on an optimistic note worth discussion, the most identifiable difference between 1918 and present day is our technology sector, and the ability to act as a worldwide unit larger than could have ever been possible prior to present day. We have been given a Ferrari in the world of medical advancement, capable of information analytics so rapid that it can surpass real-time spread of epidemics and potentially save countless people. When this is ethically and accurately cared for, it can breed trust within the community. This trust can lead to a global response on a unified front. We have never been more connected than we are now, and that may be what it takes to take on a disastrous illness such as this. We have the capability to respond, and it is imperative that we take on this responsibility.

ALSO BY WAR HISTORY JOURNALS

MONGOOSE BRAVO: VIETNAM: A TIME OF REFLECTION OVER EVENTS SO LONG AGO

"A frank, real, memoir" – Reviewer

Uncover the gritty, real-life story of a Vietnam combat veteran.

With an engaging and authentic retelling of his experiences as an infantry soldier of the B Co., 1/5th 1st Cavalry Division in the Vietnam War, this gripping account details the life and struggles of war in a strange and foreign country.

WORLD AT WAR: UNFORGETTABLE TALES FROM THE FIRST AND SECOND WORLD WARS

"True Stories of Endurance, Horror and Beautiful Human Beings." – Reviewer

Haunting Truths We Must Never Forget.

Follow in the footsteps of the British, German and American servicemen as they detail the life and struggles of war in mysterious and foreign countries. Uncover their mesmerizing, realistic stories of combat, courage, and distress in readable and balanced stories told from the front lines.

This book brings you firsthand accounts of combat and brotherhood, of captivity and redemption, and the aftermath of wars that left no community unscathed in the world. These stories have everything from spies and snipers to submarines and air raids. A great book for anyone who wants to learn what it was like during the world war conflicts between 1914-1945.

BROKEN WINGS: WWI FIGHTER ACE'S STORY OF ESCAPE AND
SURVIVAL

*"A masterfully told story of triumph and redemption in a powerfully
drawn survival epic."* – Reviewer

Hero WWI Fighter Pilot Shot Down and Captured.

With an engaging and authentic retelling of his experiences as an
escaped prisoner of war, this gripping account details the life and
struggles of a captured pilot in 1917 war-torn Europe.

Lieutenant John Ryan couldn't wait to see action in WWI. He
joined up with the British colors out of Canada. As one of several
American pilots in the Royal Flying Corps before the US joined
the war, he earned his wings and became an Ace through fierce air
battles over the skies of Germany.